Other titles by Kath Melia

Nursing Ethics (with I. E. Thompson and K. M. Boyd)
Learning and Working: the occupational socialization of nurses

EVERYDAY NURSING ETHICS

KATH M. MELIA
B.Nurs. (Manc.), Ph.D.

MACMILLAN

First published 1989

Published by
MACMILLAN EDUCATION LTD
Houndmills, Basingstoke, Hampshire RG21 2XS
and London
Companies and representatives
throughout the world

Typeset by Wessex Typesetters
(Division of The Eastern Press Ltd)
Frome, Somerset

Printed in Hong Kong

British Library Cataloguing in Publication Data
Melia, Kath M.
Everyday nursing ethics.
1. Medicine. Nursing. Ethical aspects
I. Title
174'.2
ISBN 0–333–47152–0

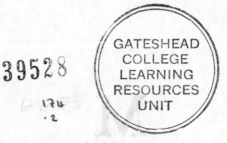

CONTENTS

ACKNOWLEDGEMENTS

The author and publisher wish to thank *Nursing Times* for permission to reproduce articles which appeared originally in the journal within the Series 'Everyday Ethics for Nurses'.

PREFACE

As a practical introduction to nursing ethics *Everyday Nursing Ethics* is for both nursing students and qualified nurses. It takes a case-based approach to a range of issues which confront all nurses and challenges them to think about the ethical dimension of their work. Nurses working in daily clinical contact with patients should be able to identify with at least some of the cases and so be able to use the book within their practice rather than viewing ethics as some kind of ivory tower philosophical discussion which does not relate to practice. Nursing students will find the book a stimulating resource which sets theory firmly into practical settings.

Each chapter deals with an important issue. In a brief and readable way it introduces the relevant ethical theory which is then developed so that the reader can build up an understanding of the different arguments that have been put forward by key moral philosophers in order to justify particular moral stances. These arguments are illustrated by relating them directly to a case so that the reader can see how ethical debate works. The cases quoted are, for the most part, not the dramatic ethical dilemmas; rather they are about the everyday realities which nurses face when ethical decisions are being taken or have been taken. So the book is not about 'do we turn off the machine?' but more about 'what are the implications for nurses in a personal and professional sense when the machine is turned off?'

It is important to realise that the book is *not* about deciding what is right and wrong in nursing practice. Each of us is entitled to a position and so no one should be excluded from voicing an opinion – this is the essence of true ethical debate. However, discussion is likely to be more constructive if we have a clear idea about how to put arguments together, and an insight into the reasoning behind the moral positions we take.

The book is designed for use by individual nurses or as a basis for ward or classroom-based group discussion. Each chapter includes points for discussion; an annotated bibliography at the end of the book will enable readers to take the issues further.

INTRODUCTION

Writings on things ethical are becoming popular both in the general and the nursing press. Whether this interest in moral issues would have reached its zenith without advances in medical technology, cutbacks in the health service, violence against women and children and, of course, the arrival of AIDS, remains one of life's imponderables. Whatever the cause, nurses are becoming increasingly interested in the ethical dimension of their care, and rightly so.

Moral problems and ethical issues need not always be of dilemma proportions. In day-to-day nursing there are occasions when we have to make decisions which have moral overtones. We make choices, for instance, not only about where to put material resources but also resources in the form of ourselves, our time and our effort. Moral dilemmas of the 'do or die' variety help us to focus upon the moral choices we must make, and so debating ethical dilemmas is a useful exercise. We should not, however, allow the big dilemmas to detract from the more routine moral choices involved in nursing.

Take for example, a simple and all too common situation – a shortage of sheets. It is 7.30 am and a ward of 30 geriatric patients has only 18 sheets for the day. The advice from the nursing officer is to 'use them sparingly'. There are clearly practical and political issues here – questions of organisation and resource allocation. Yet for those confronted with the situation there remains the question – who gets the sheets? How are decisions made? Which patients will have to manage without?

Nurses in such a situation have to make choices of a practical and moral nature – how? Beyond the who gets the sheets question is the wider issue of how should nurses react to such a shortage. One option would be to take nursing's time-honoured approach of 'coping', showing how resourceful nurses can be – but at what cost? A more radical, and personally threatening, response would be to stand out and say that patients cannot be cared for in such conditions. How far should nurses go to help shore up the system? Just what constitutes the best care of patients?

The first question we need to address is whether we should consider nursing ethics to be independent of medicine. Could nursing ethics not simply be a reflection of medical ethics? There are, of course, occasions giving rise to ethical concern that are the same for medicine, for example abortion, euthanasia, care of the mentally ill, reproductive technology, intensive care. But the difference for ethical debate lies in the way the issues present and the nature of the practical problems they bring. The medical profession is often deemed to have the last word in ethical decisions, albeit in the guise of clinical judgement, because doctors 'carry the legal can'.

Nursing's position in relation to medicine is to a large extent determined by power. This means that issues of power and control essentially define the domain of the concerns of nurses. Doctors may take decisions to discontinue care – nurses have to put that decision into practice; doctors may admit a patient on a voluntary basis, it is the nurse who has to 'keep' the patient in the ward. Nursing ethics has, then, a life of its own.

Given this state of affairs, nursing ethics should concern itself with debates which should lead us through and beyond the more publicised ethical stamping grounds of abortion and euthanasia to the twilight zone of when to tell patients the truth, what to do when you oppose a course of treatment, how to react when staffing levels force unpalatable decisions and other ethical problems that face nurses every day.

In this book we shall be looking at everyday, and some not-so-everyday, situations. The aim is to take time to consider the moral aspect of nursing work. If this sounds a bit 'ivory tower' and removed from the cut and thrust of nursing in the raw, nothing could be further from the case. Ethics, the study of morals, is very practical because decision making in health care has its moral as well as clinical, psycho-social and economic aspects. In the daily round of clinical decision making the social and economic consequences have to be considered. After all there are social relations to be maintained and budgets to be met. However, unless a major dilemma presents itself, the moral aspect is often overlooked, if not avoided. There is rarely time to step back and ask – was that fair? Was it just? Was it right?

If we were to ask such questions, how would we set about finding the answers? Consult the moral procedure book? Clearly not. While we all have our own personal morality, those involved in health care have to take that morality into a public arena and work in a professional capacity. Codes of ethics are of some help and we shall discuss these during the course of the book but codes are only part of the picture. How do we decide what is morally justifiable in our dealings with patients?

As a society, the best we can hope for is some form of moral consensus about what is acceptable behaviour and what is not. The same is true both within and between the health care professions. Such is the nature of morality that one form of moral behaviour cannot be said to be *a priori* superior or more desirable than another. Moral positions must be argued for and justified. In any case, often we will not know whether we have taken the right decision.

Discussing these matters helps us to express our feelings on moral issues and to encourage us to justify the positions we take. In everyday life we tend to take our moral stances for granted – it is wrong to steal, we should tell the truth, we should behave well towards our neighbour and so on. In other words, we do not question the basis upon which our values or principles stand.

In this book we shall look at the justification for the values we hold and at moral theory, which helps us to examine what we take for granted. Ethics is a severely practical business, for without real life situations, moral debate would be singularly sterile. The intention is, then, to centre discussion around cases and typical situations and to proceed from the practical reality to the more general discussion. Thus notions such as 'justice', 'beneficence' (duty to care), 'respect for persons', 'confidentiality' and 'rights' will be seen to be directly related to the day-to-day care of patients.

3

1

TO LIE OR
NOT TO LIE?

There are some things we take for granted which make the day-to-day business of living possible. One of them is telling the truth. No one would be so naïve as to suppose that lies, white and otherwise, are not told from time to time, but we must have some basic ground rules whereby we can expect to be dealing with the truth, until we have reason to believe otherwise. I refer here to the everyday sense of truth rather than to any philosophical notion of its nature.

Put at its simplest, we are taught from quite a young age that we should not tell lies. It is not long, however, before we discover that situations in life can often be rendered more comfortable if we tell a lie, or are, as the cabinet secretary put it, 'economical with the truth'. The same discovery is made soon after entering nursing. Any illusions nursing students may have had that patients are kept fully informed about their condition, progress and prognosis are soon dispelled.

Truth telling is a complicated business. We can often find unselfish reasons to justify not telling the truth. Nevertheless much stress is laid on honesty and to a great extent we judge those around us according to their trustworthiness. Political careers are made and broken on issues of trust.

For similar kinds of reasons, trust is important in nursing. Patients place themselves in the care of medical and nursing staff because they trust nurses and doctors.

There are occasions, however, when nurses may be tempted to be untruthful, if it makes for the smoother handling of an awkward situation. Can they really justify being less than honest with patients? Indeed are there times when nurses *should* conceal the truth from patients? Consider the examples in the case studies.

CASE STUDIES

1   During a busy medicine round a staff nurse gives the wrong drugs to one of the patients. It is a simple case of fixing the right face to the wrong name, compounded by not checking the patient's name band. After a moment's panic, the staff nurse realises that the drug was an innocent vitamin and, as the patient has not noticed, decides that a 'least said soonest mended' approach would be prudent. The incident is not reported.

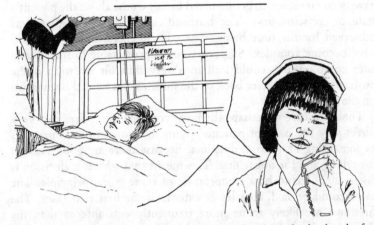

2   A third-year student speaks on the telephone to the husband of a woman who has been to theatre. It is 12 noon and she tells him that his wife is back from the theatre, conscious and comfortable. In fact she has the wrong patient in mind, the wife of the man is still in theatre. However, when the husband arrives to visit in the evening his wife is conscious, but only just. He is concerned as he had expected his wife to be brighter as she had been fully round from the anaesthetic since lunchtime. He asks the student why his wife is so drowsy. Rather than admit to the man that she gave him the wrong information, and cause him to lose faith in the hospital, she tells a few white lies about anaesthetics.

3   A patient has been given only some of the facts about his condition – he asks a student nurse if the obstruction is cancer. She knows that a decision has been taken not to tell this man the whole story, yet she feels obliged to answer him truthfully. What should she do? She says she will get sister. In doing this, she knows that she has probably increased his suspicions, and that if sister abides by the decision, he will be none the wiser.

In each of the situations a case could probably be made for telling the truth whatever the consequences, but the opposite can also be argued. In the case of the drug error it might be argued that it is always best to be honest yet, as no harm was done, the nurse had to consider whether it was worth drawing attention to her mistake and thus possibly being labelled as a careless nurse. Does the patient have a right to know what has happened to him, or would he have more peace of mind if he doesn't?

In the second case, if the mistake were admitted there would have been no reason to get involved in half truths about the patient's state of consciousness. The husband's faith in the hospital was preserved for the time being. The consequences, however, could have become complex. Surgery is an unpredictable business, and later complications could lead to a very difficult situation if the husband saw fit to refer back to the information he had been given on the day of surgery.

The third case is perhaps the most complex as it raises in a very direct way the issue of patients' rights to information. It presents as something of a moral dilemma, because there are good reasons for telling and for not telling. This means that whatever decision is taken there has to be a compromise of some moral principle. The same could be said, to a lesser extent, of the first two cases. The first two are likely to be more frequently encountered than the third, but the dramatic nature of the third makes it a useful case to debate in that it makes us sharpen up our thoughts on the whole matter of truth telling.

As nurses have to make decisions in the daily routine of nursing, without much notice or time for debate, they tend to do so according to a general notion of what seems right or suitable. If pushed to justify such decisions, which is what we begin to do when we engage in ethical debate, a nurse might justify her actions by recourse to some higher principle. For instance, in these cases it might be argued 'one should always tell the truth'; the more general principle upon which that rests is that of 'respect for persons' and their 'autonomy'.

Beauchamp and Childress[1] explain moral reasoning in terms of deliberations and justifications at different levels. First there are the particular judgements that nurses make for individual cases – to tell a patient his diagnosis. At another level there are rules which state what ought and ought not to be done; for instance, it is wrong to lie. These rules are justified by more general or fundamental principles; in the case of rules about truth telling, 'respect for persons' is the relevant principle. Finally at the highest level of abstraction, there are ethical theories which bring the principles and rules together; for example utilitarian (common good) and deontological (based on duty) theories. This kind of thinking, which looks at the principles upon which we act, sets a framework within which we can consider the nature of moral choice.

If we are to withhold the truth about diagnosis from patients there must be good reasons for doing so. It is often argued in defence of lying to patients that knowledge of the facts might actually do patients harm, or will be upsetting for them. Higgs[2] does not argue with the idea that patients may be upset by the truth, but he points out that this paternalistic, protective stance is peculiar to health care professionals. In no other walk of life, he says, would professionals regard it as their duty to suppress information simply in order to preserve happiness.

The fundamental question in all this is whether we can make a better case for not telling the truth than for telling it. The most common justification offered for lying to patients is that it is in their best interests. Hence we justify withholding diagnostic information from a patient by drawing upon the principle of 'beneficence', or a duty to care.

I said earlier that to be forced to choose between two courses of action often involves a choice between two sets of principles, thus creating a moral dilemma. In the third case arguments about respect for persons are set against those of the duty to care for patients in a way which best suits their interests.

Following this line necessarily compromises the notion of respect for persons and their autonomy. The duty to care principle leads nurses, on occasion, to take decisions out of the patient's hands and into their own. The problem here is that making decisions for patients, deciding what they should and should not be told, is undertaken in much the same way as the rest of their treatment is carried out.

In this way the infringement of a patient's rights is viewed in clinical rather than moral terms in the everyday world of nursing and medicine. Yet there are moral aspects to such decisions. This approach to care can be seen as mere benevolent paternalism – a 'father knows best' stance – which takes away the patient's capability to act as a free and autonomous individual.

This complex of issues – respect for persons, autonomy and

beneficence – is problematic, and each merits fuller discussion. In the next chapter I shall take the notions of autonomy and respect for persons a little further in the course of a discussion of artificial reproduction and the attendant issue of embryo experimentation.

It is also worth noting that partial revelation and distortion of facts can lead to difficulties at all levels in health care. The furore during the early days of the AIDS problem over the British Medical Association's advice to potential blood donors is a good example of the difficulties to which pronouncing limited truths can lead. The Blood Tranfusion Service was quick to realise that for blood supplies the implications of the BMA's statement[3] would be catastrophic – a different truth had to be told.

AREAS FOR DISCUSSION

I hope that qualified staff and students will use this book to stimulate discussion of the moral issues in nursing. The questions below do not necessarily have 'correct' answers; they are designed to focus attention on some of the moral quandaries raised by the 'should we always tell the truth?' debate. You may like to try them out on yourself and some of your colleagues.

- Are there any circumstances in which you would not tell a patient the truth in response to a straight question?
- If so, what circumstances would justify a lie, or an evasive response?
- Is there any distinction in moral terms between withholding information and deliberately misleading?
- What do you do when you disagree with medical instructions about what patients should be told?
- Can it *ever* be in a patient's best interests not to know?
- How far do nurses take away patients' rights to control their own lives and make decisions for themselves?
- Are there times when nurses really do know best?

NOTES AND REFERENCES

1. T. L. Beauchamp, J. F. Childress, *Principles of Biomedical Ethics*, 2nd edn (Oxford University Press, 1983).
2. R. Higgs, 'On telling patients the truth', in M. Lockwood, *Moral Dilemmas in Modern Medicine* (Oxford University Press, 1985).
3. The BMA's press statement placed profound restrictions on the eligibility for blood donations.

2

MEASURING FREEDOM

One of the basic assumptions we all make is that, within the limits of the law, we have freedom to act as we choose. Of course, we all have certain constraints placed on us by work, family and our social environment but, generally, we make our own decisions and act accordingly.

This freedom to act as we please is based on the idea of 'autonomy'. And autonomy depends on our capacity to think and act on the basis of our own reasoning.

In so-called free societies we value freedom and autonomy, especially when we remember those areas of the world where people cannot take their autonomy and civil liberty for granted. However, a closer look at our own society reveals that some of its citizens are more free than others.

Leaving aside prison inmates and the socially and economically disadvantaged, there are still groups who cannot exercise their free will. They are people who have to rely on others for their care and daily needs. Their personal circumstances vary widely from the severely mentally handicapped, who are incapable of reasoning, to the grossly physically disabled who are often, despite their mental alertness, 'taken over' by their carers. Between these extremes are many different circumstances and needs, and they can be found in acute and chronic care settings.

The two cases presented in this chapter are simple illustrations of the everyday constraints of hospital life which can put nurses in the position of curtailing patients' freedom. Often there is no time to consider in any great detail the infringement of patients' liberty or, indeed, to regard such incidents in that light at all. This is in part because these decisions are taken in the patients' best interests and in accordance with the nurses' duty to care. Nurses regard their

10

actions in terms of doing the best they can, rather than deliberately setting out to infringe patients' rights to autonomy.

In the case of the old lady, it is argued that the frail elderly may fall and fracture a bone and so the hospital must take action to prevent such an occurrence. The danger of falling is a fact of life for the elderly; the question is, how far should the hospital go in its efforts to maintain the safety of patients in this respect? Should all elderly patients have their activities curtailed and their lifestyles constrained to the extent that it causes distress because they *might* fracture a femur? Or is there a right to risk such a fracture? And if there is such a right, who should control the exercise of it – the nurse, the patient, or the patient's relatives?

A judgement is clearly required in every case, bearing in mind the mental and physical capacity of the patient. There are moral aspects to such judgements involving the ideas of 'beneficence' and 'non-maleficence' – doing good and doing no harm. I shall do no more than make mention of these moral principles here and return to them later.

Unfortunately, there is a tendency in institutions to fit care into a routine and to resort to general rules, and bureaucratic solutions to individual situations. Some patients' autonomy seems to be respected more readily and to a greater degree than that of others. If the old lady had been younger and had all her mental powers, or the boy had been an adult, perhaps time would have been found to meet their needs.

These are everyday, relatively trivial, examples. Yet they concern fundamental issues of freedom to choose and act.

Are there then times when nurses may ignore patients' autonomy? There will certainly be times when staff should take over a patient's autonomy in order to ensure his safety. The problem is where to draw the line. Are you always sure that it was in the patient's best interest that his will was overridden? Or did the convenience of the staff and the institution take precedence?

This leads us to ask what is it that places a moral obligation upon nursing staff to respect patients as fully autonomous persons? This may seem a dreadful question to ask, but as we shall see it is not as clear cut as it may first appear. To try to address it, let us look at an area of health care where it has been most rigorously addressed – the status of the human embryo.

The moral issues here centre around the question: 'Should the embryo be afforded the same respect as a human being?' This

11

question is especially important, as the Warnock report pointed out[1], in the light of current *in vitro* fertilisation practices which involve more embryos being produced than will be transferred to the uterus.

Among the issues most fiercely debated is the moral acceptability of allowing so called 'spare embryos' to die. The vexed questions of the moral status and rights of the embryo are inescapable. The DHSS in 1986 put out a consultation paper to assist in the drafting of legislation on human infertility services and embryo research[2] and the new legislation is now under way.

Those in favour of research do not accept that the embryo has the same full human status as a child. They argue in favour of experimentation on, and then destruction of, the embryo because this has benefits to offer mankind in infertility treatment, the study of congenital abnormalities and improvements in techniques of contraception.

Those against experimentation argue that the embryo, from conception, has the same status as a child or adult and so may not be researched upon in a way which would not only be of no benefit to it, but would lead to its eventual destruction. There is also some dispute about the clinical benefits of research on early embryos.

The debates that surround the issues of 'spare embryo' production and disposal turn on the question of 'what is a person?' The British philosopher John Locke defined a person as 'a thinking intelligent being that has reason and reflection and can consider itself as itself, the same thinking thing, in different times and places'.[3]

This definition clearly leaves room for debate about whether different members of the human species need to be accorded full rights as 'persons'. Embryos, foetuses and very young infants and people with severe brain damage would all fall outside it. In drawing these distinctions we begin to see where making decisions about who has and who has not the right to be treated as a fully autonomous person might lead.

It also allows us to think about the patients in our care who might not fulfil Locke's qualification as a person, yet for whom we feel morally obliged to care, but to whose autonomy we may give little thought. These are the patients who perhaps make us feel uncomfortable because we have difficulty in thinking about them in the same way that we regard ourselves. We plainly cannot put these patients, for instance those who are completely demented and aggressive, in the same category as some would put the spare embryo; that is, less than human and therefore disposable.

The philosopher Immanuel Kant argued for the principle of 'respect for persons'. He started with the premise that rational beings will be bound by what he calls the 'supreme moral law', and that we should always act in such a way that our actions could be universally applicable to others.

Kant argued that people have an inherent moral worth which makes it necessary for us to treat each other as ends in ourselves, and not simply as a means to an end. This 'do as you would be done by' maxim is common to many philosophical postions; for instance, the Golden Rule of Moses: 'Do unto others as we would have them do unto us.' Kant stressed the point that, however worthwhile the consequence of an action might be, people had to be treated as ends in themselves and that any other kind of approach was not morally acceptable.

Kant's ideas may give us some guidance as to how to behave towards people, but in the collective setting of health care, just how helpful is he in our day-to-day decision-making? The idea that our actions should be universally applicable is perhaps of the most practical use in our moral deliberations, along with the 'treat others as you would have them treat you' maxim.

Yet, as we have seen, there will be occasions where equal treatment is not deemed to be right for that circumstance. Kant's ethics leave us with some difficult questions. Do some patients have less right to our respect because they are not 'rational beings'?

Raanan Gillon suggests that this is the case, both philosophically and in fact[4]. He says: 'The idea that a single living human being starts its existence not being a person, develops into a person, and then at some stage may stop being a person, while remaining a living human being seems to be intuitively plausible, both as an account of what happens and also as a basis for at least some sorts of important moral distinction.' The notion of 'brain death' clearly supports this view.

The principle of 'respect for persons' helps us to sharpen up our thinking about how we act towards patients. In principle, the idea of each person being autonomous and having a right to life is a good one. In practice, however, there are difficulties.

Sometimes scarce resources do not allow provision of the care which would be in the patient's best interests. In emergency situations, where the patient is seriously ill or unconscious, he is unable to exercise autonomy. The interests of one patient may

CASE STUDIES

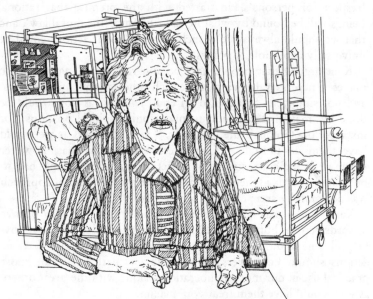

1   A first-year nursing student is working with a nursing auxiliary on a busy geriatric ward. The elderly demented lady whom they have just got out of bed, dressed and sat in her chair, asks if she can go to the balcony to see the garden. She starts to cry and tries to get up by herself. The auxiliary, securing the old lady into her chair by fixing the table in place, says to the student: 'She always asks that, she'll fall if we leave her and we haven't got time to stay.' This is in fact the case, the lady has made the same request each morning for the past few months and the ward is understaffed. What else could they do? Does the old lady really mind sitting in her chair? Has she the right to take up any more of their time at the expense of other patients? Whatever the case, the old lady is upset and has not exercised her autonomy.

2   Another example concerns a ten-year-old boy with heart arrhythmia who is being nursed in an adult ITU. He asks to be allowed to go to the hospital shop for a change of scene and to buy a comic. The staff are too busy to take him and cannot let him go alone. He complains for the rest of the morning, making everyone feel guilty. Even though he knows that the decision was made on the basis of necessity and in his own best interests, he still felt that he was being restricted unfairly.

conflict with those of another and questions of justice then arise.

I have considered autonomy and respect for persons in a general way and focused on the early stages of life. Keeping to these principles presents problems at the end of life too. In the next chapter I shall consider some of these issues in the light of the principle of 'beneficence' – doing good for others.

AREAS FOR DISCUSSION

- Discuss the limits on your own freedom – do you decide what these limits are or are they imposed from outside?
- Do you accept that it is right to restrict a patient's freedom 'in his own best interests' and, if so, who should decide what are his best interests?
- Is it right to differentiate between patients when considering autonomy? Does an embryo have the same rights as a child, or a demented old lady the same rights as a young man?
- Can you think of a situation where a patient's autonomy was unnecessarily restricted? What makes cases like these different from those where restrictions were justified?
- Does it help having some insight into the moral dimension in all this, or are time and pressure of work the real masters? Or are they just excuses?

NOTES AND REFERENCES

1. *Report of the committee of inquiry into human fertilisation and embryology* (Warnock report) (London: HMSO, 1984).
2. *Legislation on human infertility services and embryo research: a consultation paper* (London: HMSO Cm 46, 1986)
3. J. Locke, 'Essay concerning human understanding', in J. Perry, *Personal Identity* (University of California Press, 1975).
4. R. Gillon, *Philosophical Medical Ethics* (London: John Wiley, 1986).

3

CRUEL TO BE KIND?

Nurses and doctors have long taken the view that they know best how to treat and care for patients. Indeed, by the nature of the work they do doctors and nurses have a duty to care for their patients. A patient has to be able to trust his health care professionals and to presume that they will act in ways which serve his needs.

In turn, professionals expect that they will be trusted by patients. Such is the strength of the obligation that doctors and nurses have to provide care that they extend the obligation beyond their professional hours. Doctors and nurses may be called on at public events if there is an accident or someone is taken ill. As Raanon Gillon[1] points out, we do not expect to hear calls across public address systems for any architects in the room to go to reception; and if such a request was made, an architect would not feel the slightest obligation to respond. It is the duty to care which sets health professionals apart and places certain obligations upon them.

Relationships between hospital nurses and doctors and their patients are influenced by the fact that they work in institutions and are bound both by the rules governing the hospital and by professional codes of conduct and ethics. I shall return to these features of the patient–professional relationship. I mention them here simply to highlight their importance in the context of the duty to care. In other words, when carrying out their duties, nurses and doctors have to take into account rather more than the immediate demands of their individual patients.

At the heart of this duty to care is the premise that health professionals should 'do good' and 'do no harm'. The International Council of Nurses' Code for Nurses[2] states 'the fundamental responsibility of the nurse is fourfold: to promote health; to prevent illness; to restore health and to alleviate suffering.' In the Hippocratic

16

Oath, a doctor promises that the treatments adopted 'shall be for the benefit of the patient according to my ability and judgement and not for their hurt or for any wrong.'

The philosophical terms used for this 'doing good' and 'doing no harm' are beneficence and non-maleficence respectively. Beneficence entails positive action. Beauchamp and Childress say there are three 'oughts' involved in beneficence[3]. These are: to prevent evil or harm, to remove evil or harm and to do or promote good. Non-maleficence entails not inflicting evil or harm, in other words not doing that which is bad. We can see that these four elements of beneficence and non-maleficence relate directly to the ICN Code.

Like motherhood and apple pie, beneficence is universally welcomed as 'a good thing', but in practice it is rather more problematic. Who is to say what is in the patient's best interests? Is it always possible to sort out the harm from the good? Does the old adage that you 'have to be cruel to be kind' have a place in all this? To put it bluntly, how do we know what might, from the patient's viewpoint, do more harm than good? Are there ever times when nurses would feel that it is their duty to care for a patient against his wishes? How far should we go in our attempts to treat patients in their own interests?

Clearly in this kind of discussion we need to bear in mind on the one hand the notion of autonomy and, on the other, benevolent paternalism, or 'nurse knows best' in the most positive sense of that term.

Let us first consider the idea of doing good and not doing harm in the practical situations proposed in the case studies.

In the first case the student nurse sees her duty to care in a fairly simplistic sense; that is, she aims to bring comfort to the old lady. In fact her view of the situation is not very far removed from that of the elderly lady herself. The student knows the sister has other considerations in mind – the recovery of movement and a capacity for more independence in the patient. She also knows that if the patient is treated in this entirely passive way, there is a likelihood not only that she will fail to improve, but that her condition will worsen. Thus, we have a duty to prevent harm as well as to do good. The problem is that in trying to balance the two to the satisfaction of the nursing staff's understanding of their duty to care, the patient's wishes are left out of the count.

In the second case, the patient's nutrition presents some of the same problems. The harm that ensues from not caring for the

17

patient, in this instance not feeding him, has to be set against the good that might come from adhering to his wishes. The old man may simply have had enough and be content to let nature take its course. This seems to be the premise upon which the charge nurse made the decision not to press food on the old man. A patient's refusal to eat presents singularly difficult conflicts for nurses.

The question of whether it is sometimes right to allow a patient to starve himself is plainly emotive. There are legal implications and there may be fears that nurses would be liable to charges of negligence. And apart from all this, it goes against all the instincts of caring to leave someone without food. Yet, the spectacle of a patient being fed against his will and the accompanying loss of dignity is not one which many nurses relish.

It is worth noting too that the refusal to eat only moves into the moral arena because the patient is in hospital. This is partly because of the professional obligation to care and partly because the health authority has a vicarious responsibility for the patient. To choose not to eat for a few days at home is a matter of free choice, in hospital this freedom is curtailed.

The question of whether or not it is doing good to feed the old man thus has to be tempered with considerations of non-maleficence – that is not doing him harm. If we judge the harm – his distress and discomfort at being fed – is so great that it outweighs the good (that is, seeing that he has adequate nutrition) then the charge nurse's course of action was more appropriate than that of the staff nurse. If in this situation you were to ask yourself: 'How do I justify feeding or not feeding this old man?' you would, in a very practical sense, be right in the middle of a debate about beneficence and non-maleficence.

The third case, about the lady who had a history of coronary heart disease, confronts the issue of deciding what the patient's best interests are. What would constitute beneficence in this situation? The nurses, in asking for a policy on resuscitation were, wittingly or otherwise, asking for a decision to be taken; a decision which involved weighing the merits of intervention and its possible attendant good against the harm that might come from such an action.

The question of whether or not to resuscitate arises because the patient is in hospital. While acknowledging that if the old lady had been in the street, any competent first-aider might have put her through the same ordeal, the hospital orientation to saving life makes resuscitation much more likely. The question of when it is appropriate to resuscitate is always vexed and it is particularly so with elderly people. Nurses quite reasonably like to have clear instructions about whether to resuscitate. Doctors equally understandably, are often reluctant to write the *not for resuscitation* 'sentence' into the notes. Yet 'hurrying slowly' and hoping for the best is not really good enough. Doctors and nurses are generally understood to be in the business of saving and preserving lives. Public trust is placed in them for that reason.

On the whole preserving life is considered to be a good thing although individual professional judgements are clearly made for each case. The public might find entering a hospital even more traumatic if they felt that 'not for resuscitation' orders were common. On the other hand, that knowledge might well be of great comfort to many, including the frail elderly and the chronic sick. The oft heard complaint that 'no-one dies any more – they arrest!' needs to be taken seriously.

To an extent, then, hospitalisation itself creates some of the dilemmas faced by nurses when they consider what is good for their patients. That professionals must work according to their professional organisation's rules and their oaths and codes limit their range of options. In terms of protecting society as a whole this is clearly a good thing. The trouble with broad and general rules, like beneficence, is that when it comes down to individual cases and situations, problems emerge that cannot always be solved by recourse to the general rule.

In short, there are institutional and professional constraints placed on the notion of beneficence. The good that we hope to do our patients has to be negotiated within these constraints. In obeying the duty to care, the nurse may take decisions on the patient's behalf which, if the patient were left to himself, he would not go along with. This could be said to be the down side of placing trust in professionals.

The good done by professionals is ultimately judged by weighing it against the harm that may result from the treatments and care chosen. This kind of risk/harm versus benefit equation has to be worked out all the time in health care, both with individual patients and on a larger scale. Current debate about the merits of testing, or even blind screening, for the AIDS virus is a crucial case in point.

CASE STUDIES

1 An elderly woman has sustained a stroke, and is severely incapacitated. Her care consists mainly of a rehabilitation programme by which the nurses are required to ensure that she does as much as possible for herself. This means that the old lady spends a good part of her day struggling to dress and feed herself: she rarely looks well turned out and often her food gets cold. A student nurse caring for her one morning decides to assist her in these activities to the point where the patient has to do very little. The elderly lady is extremely grateful and tells the student that she has not been so well looked after for a long time and says that she will make a special point of telling sister. The student is pleased to have brought pleasure to the patient but is aware that the sister will not view the care that she has given in the same positive light as the patient did. What should she do next time she cares for this patient?

2 An 80-year-old man recovering from bronchitis says that he does not feel like eating and that he is quite happy to be left to rest. The charge nurse thinks that he should be given drinks only and tells the nurses not to press food upon the old man. The next day a staff nurse takes over the ward. She says that he only needs encouragement to resume eating and insists that the student attempts to feed him. The old man is very distressed by this and the student nurse feels that she should not have been asked to do it against his will. The staff nurse justifies her orders saying that the nurses have a duty to feed him in order that he does not deteriorate.

3 A frail lady in her seventies is admitted to an acute medical ward after falling at home. She has a history of coronary heart disease and feels that her 'time has come'. The nursing staff want the medical staff to come to a decision about what is to be done if she has a further coronary. The medical staff give a 'wait and see' response. The lady weakens over the next few days and while she is being bathed one morning she becomes breathless. Over the next hour she becomes very drowsy and no pulse can be found. As there are no specific instructions to the contrary she is resuscitated but dies. The nurses are angry because they would have liked to have spared her an undignified death. The doctors think that the nurses' demand for written instructions not to resuscitate are not realistic in every case.

AREAS FOR DISCUSSION

- Are there ever occasions when nurses should put the patient's wishes before his well-being?
- Are nurses justified in making decisions for patients just because they have been admitted to hospital?
- Do the codes of ethics help in making day-to-day practical decisions about how you care for patients?
- How reasonable is it to expect always to have a written policy on resuscitation? Do nurses expect too much from doctors in this difficult area?
- Is the notion of beneficence of any use in the cut and thrust of daily nursing care? Or are organisational rules and ethical codes all?

NOTES AND REFERENCES

1. R. Gillon, *Philosophical Medical Ethics* (London: John Wiley, 1986).
2. International Council of Nurses 'Ethical concepts applied to nursing', *Code for Nurses* (Geneva: ICN, 1973).
3. T. L. Beauchamp, J. F. Childress, *Principles of Biomedical Ethics*, 2nd edn (Oxford University Press, 1983).

4

WHOSE MORALS ARE THEY, ANYWAY?

Today patients are more aware of their rights and health care professionals have had to take notice. Some argue that they have not taken enough notice, failing to create a consumer-driven health service. One result of all this may be that patients feel able to demand more of professionals and even to demand that which professionals are unable or unwilling to provide.

These demands may be rather more problematic than those for out-of-hours visiting, or watching a late night film after ward lights are out. They may be requests which put the nurses into a quandary.

Patients do make demands of nursing and medical staff which, for a variety of reasons, the professionals do not wish to meet. Health care professionals have to make judgements about what constitutes the best care of patients. These professional judgements often contain moral judgements and lead us into ethical debate.

In the last chapter we looked at the ideas of beneficence and non-maleficence in some fairly common situations. We concluded that nurses and doctors have to follow professional codes and, on the patient's behalf, arrive at a course of action which balances good and harm.

One of the problems in this is that actions which the professional sees as right and good may not be viewed in the same way by the patient. In this chapter, I want to concentrate on some more unusual examples which may help to sharpen up some of our thinking in this area.

The examples here raise complex emotional issues and it may help if we consider morality in two ways – professional morality and personal morality. They also raise the question of rights, and we shall return to this later.

Health care professionals, by and large, enjoy the trust of society. It is widely assumed that they will operate according to the wishes and values of the society they serve. And, on the whole, the professional values and moral standing of nurses and doctors probably do reflect those of society. Of course, in reality it is not so clear cut, but in a democratic society it may be reasonable to make this assumption.

At the same time, society and professions are made up of individuals and among individuals there will be differences in moral positions. Thus, just as an individual may hold a view which is at odds with most of society, so a nurse may find herself out of moral step with her profession.

For the sake of argument let us assume that professional morality reflects the moral position taken by society. In our first example, John is asking the nurse to do something which goes against her professional morality, and indeed, goes against the long standing view held by society in general that suicide is wrong. And yet, at a personal level, that nurse could justify helping him, given what she sees as his right to choose.

Professionals, then, do become caught up at a personal as well as professional level. And where there is a division of opinion, it will not necessarily be a simple split with the patient asking for a 'deviant' service (like euthanasia, or help in surrogacy) while the professional strives to uphold society's values. Experience suggests that it will often be more complicated and moral choices will be influenced by both professional and personal considerations. Nurses are just as likely as patients to take a 'minority' view and go against the main leanings of society and their profession. The difference is that, as health care professionals, nurses have to answer to society and their profession as well as to their own consciences.

The result of all this may be that alliances will form between groups or individuals within the professions and groups in society. So we find, for example, that the medical scientists and practitioners responsible for the advances in reproductive technology are allied with infertile couples, forming a lobby which may not have the support of the wider society or even of most health care professionals.

The consultant obstetrician Wendy Savage stood out from her professional group and allied herself with the women in her care.

The result was a mobilisation of a large section of the medical profession and a section of the public on one side, and on the other a smaller group of like-minded health care workers and lay supporters of natural childbirth.

Nurses and doctors have to decide what to do when their personal and professional inclinations clash, and they tend to look for guidance. For this the most obvious sources are the law and professional codes of conduct and ethics.

Unfortunately, in many cases, the law is not much help; it tends to look to the professions when it is called to make judgements. When medical issues are taken to the courts for resolution, the professional definition of events is very influential. McCall Smith[2] remarked in a discussion of the legal aspects of the Royal College of Nursing's code of ethics that 'the law may ultimately be called upon to define what is acceptable practice on the part of the professions but it tends to do so on the basis of what the professions themselves suggest. The law then looks for guidance to professional consensus, while the professions naturally look to the law for a statement of what they can or cannot do'.

McCall Smith concludes that 'the promulgation of a code of professional conduct is of major legal significance, in that it can be influential in the moulding of legal attitudes.'

However, there are areas where the law can be of some help. Perhaps the most explicit guidance is to be found in the 1967 Abortion Act. A nurse or doctor can, in certain circumstances, choose to opt out of abortion practices. The conscientious objection clause is a legal recognition of personal morality, although even this does not make decisions in this area easy.

Campbell[3] suggests that we 'would respect a nurse whose conscience prevented her from taking part in abortions, yet we might equally admire the one who despite the moral conflict entailed, chose to carry on, realising that opting out put a great burden on colleagues. We recognise that people may sometimes feel obliged to remain involved in a morally ambiguous situation in order to share the difficulties with their fellow human beings rather than simply choosing the action which keeps their own moral principles intact'.

Euthanasia, in the purely legal sense, is straightforward – in other words, it is against the law. So a nurse asked by a patient to assist in ending his life can refuse and call upon the law to justify her action. Clearly, if she goes along with the patient's wishes, and is discovered, she will bring herself into the realms of the criminal law. However, the fact that there is a clear legal position does not make ethical problems go away.

John's case illustrates how a nurse can be emotionally moved to a point where she would very much like to help the patient. Part of the problem here is that the nurse, if she refuses to help, has nothing to offer. She cannot reverse the disease process, nor can she improve the quality of John's life. She is thus left feeling that she has let him down, and gone against the instincts of her own personal morality into the bargain.

Society and the professions have been reluctant to move euthanasia into the same arena as abortion and enact legislation covering practice. Yet in both cases, at a basic level, we are talking about killing. The most potent case against legalising euthanasia comes in the form of the 'slippery slope' argument. Once society gets on to that slope, so the argument runs, there is no telling where it might end.

Slippery slopes clearly have their dangers and the caution urged by the majority who oppose euthanasia has to be taken seriously. However, as Harris[4] notes, 'we do not outlaw effective contraception because we fear that to practise population control is to step onto a slope that leads inexorably to the extinction of the human race'. Perhaps by 'slippery slopes' we are ducking the issue.

Surrogacy, on the other hand, is a moral issue in the balance. There is no clear legal position save that anyone arranging a surrogate pregnancy for financial gain is acting illegally. It will be interesting to see which way the professions and society react.

Our examples have been concerned with managing personal and professional morality within legal and professional frameworks. Patients should not be dependent on the personal moral disposition of their nursing and medical staff. A far-fetched example underlines the point. If an A&E department had a large proportion of Jehovah's Witnesses on the staff, it would be bizarre to allow the judgements about transfusions to be made according to their personal morality.

This case is deliberately extreme to make the point, but there have been cases where health care professionals have brought their personal morality to bear on practice. The most celebrated was that of the late Dr Leonard Arthur, the paediatrician who was tried and acquitted of attempting to murder a Down's syndrome baby. In the next chapter I shall continue this discussion and focus on the

CASE STUDIES

1 John has multiple sclerosis and has been looked after for many years in the community. One day he asks his district nurse, whom he has known for several years, to help him take his own life. The nurse knows him quite well and has a lot of sympathy with his request. She sees nothing wrong with a person ending what has become a miserable existence. However, reluctantly she tells him that she is sorry but as a professional she cannot help him. She is acutely aware that their relationship cannot be the same again.

2 A health visitor is visiting Mary, a young mother. Mary asks her if she would be willing to help a friend to arrange a surrogate pregnancy. Mary has told her friend that the health visitor, who comes into contact with many fertile couples, many of them hard up, should be able to help. The health visitor knows this to be true. What

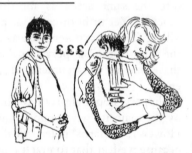

is more, she is herself unable to have children and so is particularly sympathetic. But, she is a health professional and feels that professional loyalties must come before her own personal beliefs. She, therefore, tells Mary that she cannot help her friend in this way.

3 In Brian Clark's play *Whose life is it anyway?*[1] the leading character is a sculptor who is rendered paraplegic in a car accident. He has retained all his mental faculties and has decided that he wants to be allowed to die. In one notable scene two doctors argue about his sanity. One doctor refuses to accept 'that a man of Harrison's intelligence would choose suicide'. The second points out that suicide is exactly what the sculptor has chosen, to which the first replies: 'Therefore I say he's unbalanced.' The theme of the play is the patient's right to control his life and the professional's right to save and preserve life. Its power lies in the fact that you are gradually won over to the sculptor's view and the doctors and nurses emerge as the 'bad guys'.

There is much theatrical licence in the play and few nurses would find themselves mixed up in such a dramatic conflict, but the issues are real enough.

question of nurses exploiting their professional status in an effort to further the cause of a moral pressure group.

If health care personnel have to adopt accepted professional and societal ethics and not act personally, perhaps patients too should recognise that there are limits to the demands they should make. The parameters of the professional morality in health care need to be made clear to all concerned.

AREAS FOR DISCUSSION

- Could you justify any outcome other than those described in the examples cited in this chapter?
- Do you accept that there is such a thing as professional morality? Can you think of any situations where your own views have conflicted with those of the profession? If so, what did you do?
- Can anyone expect nurses who have strong religious or other moral beliefs to put them to one side because they happen to conflict with society or the profession's accepted values?
- Can you envisage situations where you would do something as a private citizen which you would refuse to do as a nurse? Does this work the other way round?

NOTES AND REFERENCES

1. D. Benedictus, *Whose Life Is It Anyway?* (novel based on Brian Clark's play) (London: Sphere Books, 1981).
2. R. A. McCall Smith, 'Comments on the RCN code of professional conduct', *Journal of Medical Ethics* 3 (1976) 122.
3. A. V. Campbell, *Moral Dilemmas in Medicine*, 3rd edn (Edinburgh: Churchill Livingstone, 1984).
4. J. Harris, *The Value of Life: An Introduction to Medical Ethics* (London: Routledge & Kegan Paul, 1985).

5

BALANCE OF POWER

It has become increasingly fashionable to discuss health care in the language of rights – patients' rights, nurses' rights, the right to information, the right to choice, and so on. Rights may appeal to our libertarian instincts, but they are not without problems. Apart from anything else, they are not absolute in the sense that by claiming my rights I may well infringe yours.

In this chapter we consider one aspect of our rights – the right to take our personal beliefs and values into our nursing practice. Setting aside the wider debates about rights, let us try to deal with the question: 'Do nurses have a right to practise according to their own personal morality?'

The immediate, albeit knee-jerk, response to this question is to say – it depends. A patient may well say 'yes' of course a nurse should operate according to her own view of morality *provided* it fits my view. It is a case of irregular conjugation: I have a balanced view, you are wrong headed, he is off the wall! More seriously, when it comes to agreement about the moral principles upon which nursing care rests, society has a right to expect something rather less whimsical than the notion that moral judgement is an entirely private and individual affair.

In the last chapter we looked at the tension that can exist between professional and personal morality. The issues raised by this tension are many and varied. To some extent nurses do have the right to bring their personal morality to work – no one would want a profession whose members did not have some moral underpinning and ethical standards. On reflection, though, as we have seen, the degree to which they may do this could vary according to the moral position taken by each nurse. The public has the right to expect some uniformity from its nursing service and should not have to contend with morally capricious individuals.

While it is helpful to distinguish between professional and personal morality in debate, on the ground things look rather more complicated. This is because there are clearly relationships between the two, not least because professional morality is in many ways a bringing together of a consensus of individual moralities. Professional morality can be found in codes of ethics and represents the central moral principles upon which practice rests. This is rather like the general consensus on policy reached by any political party which contrasts with the variety of opinion that exists within it. Thus professional morality is something that members can broadly agree to, or at least agree to operate with.

Professional codes and agreed ways of behaving are evolved from the moral judgements and the moral choices which have been made by individuals over time. There is a down side to this – some positions are sometimes arrived at almost by default through a series of compromises made over time by practising nurses. Because of this haphazard development and the many pressures placed on nurses, undesirable aspects of care exist – for example, there are times when patients are not treated in a way which an ideal ethical code would dictate, yet this can be accepted as the norm.

Thus in many of our long-stay hospitals, among elderly and handicapped people we find what can only be described as second-class citizen status. This is not peculiar to health care professionals; society as a whole adopts stances towards groups which, if only by default, may come to be accepted. For instance, inner cities have homeless people, our prisons are over-crowded, children are brought up in far from ideal circumstances and alongside this we have widespread affluence and prosperity. As a society we have found a way of living with this and, while deploring it, we manage to accept that it exists.

Professional morality, then, has been and is shaped by the practices of its members through time and is the coming together of individual moralities to form some sort of consensus. Individual morality cannot be represented by or subsumed by the professional or collective morality; it has to coexist.

First, let us look at an extreme example – the trial of Dr Leonard Arthur. Our interest is not with the rights and wrongs of Dr Arthur's action, but with the rights and wrongs of the action of the member of Life. It has been argued that any differences of opinion

CASE STUDIES

1   The late Dr Leonard Arthur, consultant paediatrician, was tried for the murder of a severely handicapped Down's syndrome baby. The parents were distressed by the condition of the baby at birth and expressed the wish that efforts should not be made to save the baby's life. Dr Arthur entered in the case notes: 'The parents do not wish him to survive; nursing care only.' He prescribed morphine-type drugs to relieve the baby's distress and the baby died four days later. A member of Life working in the hospital contacted the police and alleged that the baby had been drugged, and left to die[1].

Throughout the trial the prosecution conceded that Dr Arthur's motives were of the highest order and that he had acted in what he considered to be a humane way for both baby and family. Nevertheless, they argued that doctors were not above the law. Expert medical witnesses endorsed Dr Arthur's actions and they were deemed to be within the norms of current medical practice. Dr Arthur was acquitted.

2   A student nurse with very strong Christian beliefs comes into contact with a patient, Mrs Brown, a committed atheist, who is in the terminal stages of cancer. The student nurse feels that she should have one last attempt to bring Mrs Brown to some understanding of the existence of God, so that she might have the chance to die as a Christian. So strong is the student's faith that she cannot conceive that Mrs Brown's conviction in the other direction is equally firm. The student nurse believes that it is her duty as a Christian to bring Christ into the lives of others whenever she can and she is confident she is acting in the patient's best interests.

3   A charge nurse in a paediatric ward feels that the parents of a child who is in the middle of a series of orthopaedic operations have not been given sufficient information about the child's prognosis. The parents have complained on 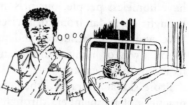 several occasions about delays, post-operative complications and what they consider to be poor nursing. The charge nurse has a poor relationship with the consultant and thinks that the nursing management does not provide him with the staffing he requires to run his ward. He also holds strong party political views on the running of the health service and so encourages the parents to write to the press and their MP.

about the care of the baby should have been made openly among professionals rather than by recourse to the police and the criminal law.

The member of Life might argue that her actions were prompted by concern over the infringement as she saw it of the child's right to live. However, she might be said to have had in mind a greater concern for the general cause of the 'Life' organisation rather than the rights and needs of the particular baby in question. After all, the doctor's decision had been taken in consultation with the parents and with the approval of the nursing staff directly involved in the care. The rights of the parents, and what was deemed to be in the best interest of the baby were infringed in the name of a wider cause championed by that individual who knew that the cause was not supported by Dr Arthur or the baby's parents.

An increasingly educated public has helped to foster pressure groups, such as Life, that represent a new lobby with which the health service has to reckon. The question here is what part should individual nurses play in these groups? If nurses cannot find a means within the health care system of having their personal views acted on, is it reasonable for them to act in a covert manner? Should they have to, or indeed do they have a right to, resort to the tactics of a mole in the organisation?

Now, let us turn to the other two cases. These raise similar points of principle for each involves personal views in a professional setting. Even if nurses are not going as far as calling the police or putting forward religious or political views in the course of their work, it is possible that their privately held beliefs and values might be brought into their work in ways that are at the very least questionable. For example, nurses may adopt a particular attitude towards a patient if they feel that the patient is in some way responsible for his condition: accidents involving drunk driving or the failure to wear a seat belt; women seeking abortion; or, of course, AIDS patients.

Nurses may also hold strong views on private medicine and so tend to be hostile towards patients occupying pay beds in NHS hospitals. The list could go on; the point is, how far is it reasonable for nurses to conduct their professional work on the basis of their personal morality?

This is a difficult area because there are causes society would want professionals to champion precisely because of their position. There may be dangers in professionals with vested interests holding certain moral positions, but an amoral profession would not only be unrealistic, it would be undesirable.

There are sound reasons for having within professions people who are prepared to make moral stands, because it is from their actions and thoughts that the moral codes are formulated through which laws are eventually shaped.

Much of the problem in all this is that the nurse–patient relationship is characterised by power. In short, the patient is a captive audience. Nurses are well placed to abuse this power if they so choose. This is as much the case if a nurse is operating according to professional morality as it is if she is putting forward personal views. The notable thing about professional morality is that it is more openly recognised and that patients, while they may not agree with the general views held by nurses, can at least recognise them for what they are.

If, on the other hand, a nurse uses her position to further some cause which nursing as a professional group does not support, then the patient may well have difficulty working out whether his interests are being served or whether they are being manipulated in the name of some other cause.

In the case of the paediatric charge nurse, the parents might feel that their own child would benefit from their efforts, whereas the nurse might have longer term goals in mind. The two outcomes are not mutually exclusive. The same applies to the boy whose pending open heart surgery became fodder for the Labour Party's 1987 election campaign – clearly, he had his own interests served, but it would be stretching the credulity of even the staunchest Labour supporter to hold that there was not a wider battle being waged.

The Dr Arthur case is complex as the parents of the Down's baby were unaware that the care of their child was being monitored by a member of staff in the hospital who espoused a cause which took exception to their decisions. There does seem to be a case for openness among professionals if we are to avoid those defensive practices which have built up in the US, due in part to legal intervention in the treatment of handicapped neonates[2].

At the centre of all this is the need to strike a balance between, on the one hand, a health service, in which all professionals are required to follow rules and regulations, and on the other, a health service in which professionals have such freedom that individual whim and sectional interests can exert influence. A service which is run according to the ethical quirks of its professionals without due regard to the views of the public it serves is clearly undesirable.

The balance, which is difficult to achieve, would seek to produce a health care service staffed by professionals who have some hand in drawing the moral codes by which they operate. This can have far-reaching consequences, for as we saw in the last chapter, professional codes of conduct can be influential in the moulding of legal attitudes.

Given the problematic nature of the power dimension getting in the way of the nurse/patient relationship and the potential for nurses' personal views getting in the way of the patient's best interests, we should perhaps place a question mark over the idea of the nurse as the patient's advocate.

AREAS FOR DISCUSSION

- Do you think that the member of Life was justified in acting as she did?
- Can professionals remain neutral or are there occasions when nurses should take up causes because the public would take more notice of a professional viewpoint?
- Should the plight of an individual patient be used to make political points?

NOTES AND REFERENCES

1. D. Brahams, M. Brahams, 'The Arthur Case – a proposal for legislation', *Journal of Medical Ethics*, 9 (1983) 12–15.
2. Institute of Medical Ethics, 'Handicapped neonates', *Bulletin Supplement*, No 5, (April 1987) 7–14.

6

WHOSE SIDE
ARE YOU ON?

Nurses have power. Like all other health care professionals, whatever strategies they use to make themselves more accessible, they cannot remove the power dimension in the professional–client relationship.

Knowledgeable professionals provide care for vulnerable patients. Nurses deal in the health arena every day and know the game and its rules. In contrast, for the patients it is an unusual, unfamiliar episode. In many ways nurses and doctors cannot win – if they make all the decisions they can be accused of paternalism, and if they leave everything to the patient they could be shirking their duty.

Most health professionals want to provide a user-friendly health service, but the complexities of NHS organisation and the imbalance of knowledge and power between professional and patient makes this difficult. This has led some observers to argue that patients need someone to help them through their encounters with the health service – someone to take *their* side.

The idea of taking different sides in health care may seem odd, but of course moral uncertainties do arise and often appear to have opposing sides. And the patient often seems to be on the losing, or at least the weaker, side. Everyone has their favourite medical experience story, just as they have their favourite British Telecom story – the main plot lines are remarkably similar, with the innocent patient/customer being given the run around by the large impersonal organisation.

We might think that having to wait half an hour or so to see a doctor or a health visitor are trivial matters. In the strictest sense they are, but these minor inconveniences serve to feed the general view among the public that health care does not come easily and has to be fought for. Perhaps this is one reason why there is now much talk of advocacy in health care.

Nurses have not been slow to stake a claim in the business. Kohnke[1] says that 'everybody talks about advocacy and seems to be doing it. The term involves such connotations as "protect" and "rights" and conveys the idea that it is something that "good guys" do'. Advocacy has to do with defending or pleading the causes of another. Kohnke argues that the nurse advocate role involves informing and supporting and she contrasts this with the lawyer as advocate. Unlike the lawyer, who presents the client's case, the nurse advocate, Kohnke says, allows the patient to make the decision, the nurse then abides by it and defends the patient's right to make it.

In many situations it would be difficult to practise a pure form of advocacy like this. The nature of the professional–patient relationship is such that advocacy is much more likely to resemble benevolent paternalism on the part of the nurse and trusting acceptance on the part of the patient. Kohnke's version of advocacy is an ideal and a somewhat naïve one at that.

Before nursing rushes down the advocacy road, we need to look at where we are going and at the legal and ethical implications. We should first ask whether nursing has a mandate to undertake the role of patient advocate. If we take a wide definition of advocacy and assume that nurses will on many occasions go beyond informing and supporting and be concerned with pleading the patient's case, we need to ask whether nurses could plead the patient's case as a barrister would plead a client's case at law.

Side-taking in a court is clear with prosecution and defence; the health care analogy is not so obvious. A patient may feel that the 'them' of the health care system are not acting in his best interests, but if he has to rely on some of 'them' taking his side he might well find that the scales are unequally tipped.

The argument for nursing taking on the patient advocate role generally involves reference to the fact that it is the nurse who spends the longest periods of time with the patient and so has a chance to build a relationship. Henderson's ideas about doing for patients that which they would do for themselves were they able, clearly suggests some notion of advocacy in the nurse's role[2]. In the first two of our examples nurses find themselves in a situation where they believe a patient is being treated inappropriately.

Both point up the difficulties of advocacy. Nurses who stand up

CASE STUDIES

1 An elderly lady, having sustained several strokes, is unconscious, incontinent and paralysed. Even though she has a very poor outlook she is being tube fed. The nurses think that the feeds are simply prolonging a life which will be of poor quality. They argue that if the old lady had a choice she would not wish to go on. On the basis that they understand the patient's position, 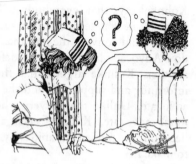 the nurses in the ward adopt the position of patient advocate and whenever the opportunity presents itself they argue that the medical staff should discontinue the calorie input and simply keep her comfortably hydrated.

2 A psychiatric patient has complained to the nursing staff that her drugs make her feel drowsy and generally unwell. The charge nurse maintains that the patient's views should be taken seriously and medication stopped. The medical staff disagree and continue to prescribe, arguing that her condition will deteriorate if medication is discontinued. The charge nurse takes a stand on the patient's behalf and refuses to administer the drugs.

3 In 1982 a Down's syndrome baby, with a gross oesophageal abnormality, was born in Bloomington Hospital, Indiana. There was a disagreement among the medical staff over treatment. One favoured surgery at another hospital while the other thought that the baby should remain in Bloomington and be made comfortable and painfree. The latter course would lead to the baby's death. The parents, when given those facts, decided in favour of allowing the baby to die. The Bloomington Hospital management called in the local judge to make a ruling. The judge found that the parents had a right to choose a recommended course of medical treatment for their child.

There followed legal wrangles involving the State Supreme Court, which upheld the first judge's decision. President Reagan responded to public pressure by ordering that the Secretary for Health and Human Services ensure that the federal laws protecting the rights of handicapped citizens were properly enforced. The law essentially states that the recipients of federal funds should not withhold benefits of services from the handicapped simply on the grounds that they are handicapped.

for what they see as the patient's rights make themselves vulnerable on two counts. First, as we have already seen, acting in the patient's best interests is not as easy as it might seem, for often one cannot be sure what the patient would think were his best interests. To take a professional judgement on the matter lays the nurse open to charges of paternalism. The patient, then, may not be happy with the nurse's actions even when they are taken in the name of advocacy. Second, the individual nurse who pleads the patient's cause may be ostracised by her colleagues. To stand up and be counted is always hard, the more so when it involves an implied criticism of colleagues.

The ethical arguments to support the advocacy role have to do with rights and obligations. A nurse who recognises what she sees as a patient's right to a certain treatment or action has a moral obligation to try to see that this is realised. Beauchamp and Childress[3] state that rights are best understood as 'justified claims that individuals and groups can make upon others and upon society'. They distinguish legal from moral rights, the former being justified by legal principles and the latter by moral principles. Rights may impose positive and negative duties on others – a patient has a right to be cared for and a right not to be harmed. Thus health care professionals have a duty to care and a duty to do no harm. Rights, then, tend to be discussed in terms of claims; this takes us into the adversarial language of the law and so to the notion of advocacy.

It is also worth bearing in mind that from the patient's standpoint, the nurse may not be the obvious candidate for the advocacy role. The main functions of the advocate which Kohnke describes, informing and supporting, could be distorted if the nurse favours a particular line of action. Because it is the nurse who has expert knowledge, the patient depends on her for the information on which to base his judgement. He is all the more vulnerable if he also has to rely on her to plead his cause.

Sometimes we forget that patients can be exposed to professional dominance by nurses, which is every bit as oppressive as medical dominance. Advocacy from this perspective starts to look like a formalised version of everyday paternalism – in other words, 'nurses and doctors know best'. In some ways this is natural, for if nurses are to make any claim to professionalism they must have something more to offer patients than they might expect from a lay person. Part of this expertise will be a capacity to make judgements about patient care; judgements which the patient may be incapable of making for himself.

If it is thought that the nurse is too much a part of the health care system to present as a plausible candidate for patients' advocate, what are the other options?

There has been an increasing tendency in the United States to turn to the legal profession – as we do in other areas of life when there is a dispute. The most publicised examples of legal involvement in medical treatment have concerned the discontinuation of life support machines, for instance, the case of the late Karen Quinlan, and the heroic treatment of handicapped neonates.

Perhaps the most dramatic example of where a legalistic approach to patients' rights might take us comes from the case which gave rise to what are known as the 'Baby Doe Guidelines' in the USA. As a result, the treatment of neonates has been affected and doctors act defensively and treat their patients according to possible legal, as well as medical, outcomes.[4]

Legalistic approaches to health care reveal the deep waters that lie under the waves of enthusiasm for advocacy. Nurses may have to live with the moral uncertainties which accompany their attempts to act in the best interests of patients when they carry out their duty to care.

To try to be a patient's friend and advocate may be to go beyond both nursing's competence and a realistic view of the nurse–patient relationship. If this is the case, then advocacy could be one bandwagon that nursing should let pass by.

AREAS FOR DISCUSSION

- Should advocacy be part of a nurse's work?
- Do you consider yourself to be a patient's advocate? If so, are there circumstances when you cannot act in that capacity?
- Would you be prepared to oppose colleagues in pursuit of what you felt was in the patient's interests?
- How do you know what is in the patient's best interests?
- Do you feel a more adversarial and legalistic approach would better serve to protect patients' rights?

NOTES AND REFERENCES

1. M. F. Kohnke, *Advocacy, risk and reality* (New York: C. V. Mosby, 1980).
2. V. Henderson, *The Nature of Nursing* (London: Collier Macmillan, 1966).
3. T. L. Beauchamp, J. F. Childress, *Principles of Biomedical Ethics*, 2nd edn (Oxford University Press, 1983).
4. H. Kuhse, P. Singer, *Should the Baby Live? The problem of handicapped infants* (Oxford University Press, 1985).

7

JUSTICE FOR ALL

As health care becomes more ambitious and medical science creates more expensive treatments, a point is reached when choices have to be made and resources put into one service at the expense of another.

Competition for a slice of the health care cake is led by the medical profession, which means that the most powerful factions and specialities have most clout. In short, the popular specialities attract most funding. Young cardiac patients, renal patients with only months to live and premature babies all attract a good press. As a result, funds are lobbied for and, more often than not, are found. In contrast, demented elderly people, those with a mental handicap and stroke victims generally attract less favourable attention and hence less finance.

In the last chapter we considered the problems surrounding the care of handicapped neonates when there is a difference of opinion about the appropriate treatment. The point was whether strenuous efforts should be made to keep alive a seriously handicapped baby if his parents requested that he should be allowed to die. We could equally question whether such a baby has a right to the resources necessary for his survival. How strong is his claim when set against the needs of the chronic sick, the elderly or people awaiting kidney transplants?

When competing needs outstrip supply, there is a certain attraction in the approach of Jeremy Bentham and John Stuart Mill. In its simplest form, their argument was that we should strive for the 'greatest happiness of the greatest number'. It would be nice to think that we could use this approach in delivering health care and thereby do the best by everyone. Yet, as Campbell has stated[1], it would be difficult to argue for preserving the lives of handicapped infants if we adopted these principles.

Ethical theories provide a framework which let us determine what we ought to do – how to act morally. Bentham and Mill's approach, known as utilitarianism, is one such theory. Its appeal is its simplicity. It deals with amounts of happiness or good.

According to this approach a moral act is one which allows for the greatest happiness or good. If there is no good to be had, the act must produce the least possible amount of harm.

There are clearly problems with a utilitarian approach when it comes to deciding what would or would not be a moral action in health care. If actions are to be judged according to the amount of happiness produced, it must be possible to calculate how much happiness will result from a particular action.

Simple utilitarian theory deals in aggregates of good and so pays little attention to the individual. Just because the cost of one heart transplant would relieve a number of people of the chronic pain from an arthritic hip, it does not detract from the relief that the single cardiac patient would obtain. What is more, he is likely to die without the transplant. Such are the problems of dealing in aggregates of happiness.

If we deal in sums of happiness we must also acknowledge who is to get into the equation. If, say, psychiatric patients were returned to large hospitals rather than being looked after by informal carers, would the relief to those carers contribute to the total sum of happiness? Would such a move produce sufficient overall happiness to enough people to justify overriding the rights of those patients?

Health care professionals rarely have to make decisions about kidneys versus hearts versus improved long-term care for the elderly. As we have seen, the internal politics of the medical profession are such that certain specialities attract resources while others remain the Cinderellas. Resources are therefore not allocated according to a master plan. Instead, allocation is a relatively *ad hoc* affair, the result of the efforts made within specialities, often by energetic individuals with a determination to develop a particular treatment.

The media also plays its part, attracted more by shroud waving than by dirty wards, or a shortage of incontinence pads. Nevertheless, nurses and doctors do face busy wards, clinics and surgeries where they have to ration their time.

In our first case study the staff nurse is under considerable pressure not to get behind with the work. If she had time to ponder

CASE STUDIES

1   In a busy medical ward, one qualified nurse, a senior student and an auxiliary are on duty. Most of the patients are elderly, recovering from strokes. There are a few younger patients who have been admitted for neurological investigations. They are anxious and constantly ask to speak to the staff nurse. She realises that these patients are anxious and that she should spend time with them. But she is equally aware of the needs of the other patients and of the fact that there will be even fewer staff on duty later in the day.

2   Nurses in an ITU have decided not to assist with a drug trial scheduled to take place on their unit. They argue that they cannot afford the time to take blood samples, to administer the drug according to a complicated schedule and to cope with the side-effects. The nurses recognise that the trial may bring a greater good for a wide range of future patients, but justify their decision in terms of wanting to meet fully the needs of their existing patients.

3   A rather disturbed girl, with very vague gastric symptoms, is admitted to a busy surgical ward because there are no other beds in the hospital. The staff nurse spends most of the evening attending to this rather manipulative patient. The staff nurse is aware that, because of this, she is not giving the other patients the attention that they deserve. When the night staff come on duty she tells them that she thinks the girl is attention seeking and suggests that they give their time to the rest of the ward. All that night the staff nurse is preoccupied with the worry that the girl might 'do something silly', and that she had been wrong to 'favour' the majority of patients at the possible expense of one patient's well being.

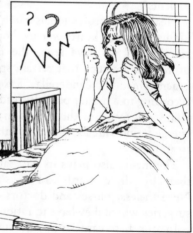

on her situation, she might see that she has to come to some decision about how to divide her time in order to try to meet the demands made upon it. She probably does not have enough time and somehow has to decide how to ration it.

In trying to meet as many needs as possible, the nurses in the second example may think along utilitarian lines – trying to do the greatest good to the largest number of patients but in the end the rights of the patients in that unit prevailed.

Perhaps we should consider again the idea of justice. Campbell argues that justice seems to contain an overriding obligation to respect the rights of individuals in cases where ignoring these rights would seem to be much more advantageous to society as a whole. It appears, then, that in some way many people feel that individual rights must come first, even if the greatest good for the greatest number is not achieved.

In the third case the doubts of the staff nurse stem from her overriding duty to respect individuals and to see that some justice is done. That is to say, she recognised that the girl's needs had to be met, even if the overall result was to compromise care for the rest of the ward. A straight utilitarian line (greatest good for the greatest number) would not pay so much heed to one individual.

In none of these three cases does the simple greatest good for the greatest number formula seem to work. Trying to meet competing needs involves some notion of distributing resources in a fair way. Aristotle[2] had an answer for this in his principle of justice. This states that equals should be treated equally and unequals unequally in proportion to their inequality. In other words, justice does not involve the equal distribution of time and care, or any other resource, to all patients. The resources have to be matched to individual needs if the allocation is to be fair or just.

There are those who suggest that medical ethics 'should have no truck with justice'. Those holding this view prefer to follow the Hippocratic obligation to do the best for each patient, arguing that if doctors temper their care for one patient with considerations about the welfare of others, that obligation cannot be filled.

Gillon[3] rejects this, arguing instead that if medicine does not concern itself with justice, someone else will. This undoubtedly applies to nursing as well. The idea that nurses and doctors need not concern themselves with justice is untenable because in everyday practice they face competing claims for scarce resources and have to make decisions as to how to proceed.

Justice appears to offer a more helpful, though complex, approach to the problems we have in trying to meet conflicting claims on our time and on health resources generally. It is worth thinking about as a basis for nurse action.

Nurses are exhorted, in a generalised and often emotional way, to care for patients while at the same time they have to make decisions about rationing that care. The decisions that nurses make about distributing their time among patients are partly clinical and partly moral judgements. A professional nursing service must make those decisions on the basis of nursing knowledge, not on some generalised emotive caring ethic.

Trained nurses are expensive and it follows that society has a right to expect that their judgements will be based upon something rather more durable than the altruism that guides lay carers.

Professional nursing decisions made by an appeal to justice should, in the long run, carry more weight than 'just doing the best we can'. Such an approach may eventually serve to remove some of the inequalities in health care – inequalities that have come about through the 'he who shouts loudest gets the most' way of allocating resources.

AREAS FOR DISCUSSION

- How do you decide how best to spread your time among a ward full of patients?
- Is it possible to weigh the interests of one patient against those of another?
- Do nurses have a primary responsibility for their own patients or should they take a wider view?
- Can you simply care for your patients whatever the cost, or should you be thinking along utilitarian lines by considering the greatest good for the greatest number?

NOTES AND REFERENCES

1. A. V. Campbell, *Moral Dilemmas in Medicine*, 3rd edn (Edinburgh: Churchill Livingstone, 1984).
2. Aristotle, *Nicomachean Ethics*, Book 5.
3. R. Gillon, *Philosophical Medical Ethics* (London: John Wiley, 1986).

8

THE SEARCH FOR OBJECTIVITY

In the last chapter we considered the ideas of utilitarianism and questioned whether they had anything to offer when making decisions about the allocation of scarce resources. On the whole we found that it was not helpful to try to decide morality on the basis of the overall amount of good produced. We seem to have an overriding obligation to consider individual needs, even if they are met at the expense of the interests of the majority.

This does not mean that utilitarianism is of no help – far from it. As Campbell[1] points out, it merits consideration because it acts as a 'good corrective to personal bias and idealistic mouthing of principles'. Whenever we discuss morals we tend to bring in our personal bias and anything that brings balance into moral reasoning can only help.

One of the attractions of utilitarianism is that it appears to introduce some objectivity. It moves us away from the 'I think that is right because I think that is right' position. It is difficult for me to argue that I am right and that my position is more reasonable than yours if my only argument is that I judge the action to be right because I know it is what I want to do. Utilitarianism moves us away from such an individual and subjective approach – it challenges the idea that only individuals can make decisions about right and wrong according to their consciences.

In the first case study in this chapter, the staff nurse has a number of options, one of which would be to tell Michael the facts of his case. Such a decision would, by and large, be made on the basis of her personal judgement about the case. She could, of course, mount various arguments about it being in his best interests to know, but on the bottom line her judgement about that cannot be said to be any more or any less valid than the doctor's. We might argue that Michael's wife is in a better position to judge than the nurse or the doctor, but even that would be to deny Michael's autonomy.

It all boils down, then, to a matter of judgement based on the staff nurse's sense of what *she* ought to do. And what this staff nurse thinks she ought to do will differ from what another nurse thinks she ought to do. Faced with the capricious nature of this kind of moral choice, it is small wonder that people look for some kind of objective moral guidance.

Utilitarian ideas offer some objectivity where other theories based on individual conscience do not.

It is worth looking at these individual conscience theories to set the more objective approaches into context. Campbell[1] says that 'most people if asked what they would do in a situation of moral uncertainty, are likely to refer to the notion of the guidance of conscience'. Conscience, he argues is 'thought of as a kind of inner voice or authority warning against wrongdoing and creating remorse when the warnings have been disregarded'. We invest our consciences with considerable authority whether or not we believe in a God.

Campbell discusses the theory of conscience which was elaborated by Butler[2] who said that obeying a conscience is part of what it means to be human. Briefly stated, Butler's theory goes like this – our motives for action involve what he calls 'particular passions and affections', 'rational calculating principles' and 'conscience'. Particular passions include our basic drives and emotional reactions like hunger or sex, fear or anger. What Butler calls 'rational calculating principles' operate to allow us to plan and assess the possible consequences of our impulses. Butler describes two such principles which serve to control the 'particular passions', namely, the principle of 'cool self love' and that of 'benevolence'. The former considers one's own happiness while the latter deals with the happiness of others.

Campbell's practical illustration of this cannot be bettered. He says that junior nurses and medical students are often overtaken by a natural reaction to human grief and suffering, that is by an 'overwhelming feeling of pity or sympathy for particular patients, which can make it extremely difficult to offer a consistent pattern of professional medical or nursing care'. They are advised by more experienced members of the profession not to get 'over involved'.

Campbell says that however 'professional' a student learns to

CASE STUDIES

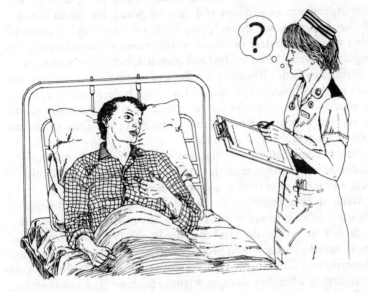

1   Michael is having haematological investigations. He calls over the staff nurse and asks her point blank if he has leukaemia. She knows that he has but she also knows that the physician after consultation with Michael's wife has decided not to tell him yet. They have decided instead to let Michael assume that he has some form of anaemia.

2   John, a patient in a psychiatric unit, has been diagnosed as manic depressive. During a period of stability he decided that he wanted to take his own life rather than face the future as a manic depressive with its distressing and debilitating mood swings. The nurses caring for John know that they have to watch him closely when he is depressed. They know that they cannot relieve his problem, but at the same time they cannot help him to do what he most wants to do – to assist suicide – although some may wish to argue that case. Instead they are obliged to ensure that John's life continues, a life that they know he has judged not to be worth living.

None of the nurses looking after John can justify their actions in terms of 'the patient's best interest' as would be the case with more tractable conditions, for they are acutely aware that his real wish is to die.

47

become, some emotional involvement with the patient's suffering will remain. This mixture of rational and emotional elements is precisely what Butler is talking about when he speaks of the interdependence of passions and rational principles. 'Both because of the student's own career plans (cool self love) and because of what will be genuinely beneficial to the patients (benevolence), the impulses have to be controlled and directed, but not cancelled out.'

Butler saw little difficulty with these two principles as he believed that, on the whole, people sought their own happiness through that of others. When there is no clear idea of what the right action should be, then conscience should come into play. Butler believed conscience was the final arbiter.

But, as Campbell argues, 'the crux of the difficulty lies in Butler's confident assumption that the individual's conscience will give a clear and inerrant answer to all moral dilemmas'.

What if two individuals' consciences come up with different answers? Who is to say which is right? The nurses who complained to an MP about the doctors' conduct in the 1987 Cleveland child abuse investigations would probably own to being guided by their consciences. Likewise, the consultants in the dispute doubtless acted according to what they thought ought to be done. The shortcomings of the individual conscience theory make it clear, then, why utilitarian ideas have some appeal.

An alternative to both is to look for something rather more absolutist – fundamental principles upon which decisions can be based. We have already seen moral laws in Kant's writings (for example, the universally applicable 'supreme, moral law' which takes a 'do unto others as you would have them do unto you' line).

The idea of natural law has been explored since Greek times[3,4,5].

The ideas of natural law are bound up with notions of a divine law, or as Campbell puts it, natural rights are thought to be generated by the law of nature. 'Natural law is regarded as that which delineates the true, or divinely intended, end of man.' By doing good (natural acts) and avoiding bad (unnatural acts) we become fully human.

All this has a 'so far so good' ring about it, for as Campbell argues, beyond this broad statement things get more difficult. When it comes to particular situations how are we to know what is good and natural and what is bad and unnatural? Are suicide, birth control and sexual intercourse outside marriage unnatural? The point at issue here is not whether these actions are wrong, but rather that a simple appeal to 'natural law' will not help to settle the question.

We are thus forced to conclude that 'natural laws', because they rest on beliefs, are not quite as rational and objective as they may first appear. Knowing that universal principles are hard to come by is of little comfort to nurses faced with moral dilemmas every day. However, there is a lot to be said for frank discussion among colleagues of their difficulties. We all tend to imagine that our colleagues have resolved the moral difficulties and that we are alone in our doubt – this is seldom the case and it is worth bringing our problems out into the open for discussion.

So far, we have pointed to the shortcomings of individual conscience, utilitarian ideas and natural law. It is as well to recognise that there are times when we are thrown back on our own consciences, however unsatisfactory or disconcerting that may be. Some testing out of the workings of our consciences through discussion could be worthwhile.

In our second case study we have a situation where the issue is not so much what is the right action to take, but where the action taken produces discomfort and moral uncertainty.

John's nurses have to decide how closely to observe him. They have to weigh up their legal and professional responsibility, his wishes and the dictates of their own consciences. Most of us can have little real understanding of deep depression. In a singularly frank account of a depressive illness an experienced psychiatric nurse summed up her feelings in the title of the paper 'There won't be a next time'[6]. She concluded from this personal experience that there are times and circumstances when 'suicide is a proper and desirable way out'.

The case of the manic depressive may not present as an immediately dramatic dilemma, but it does confront nurses with an uncomfortable situation, and day by day they have to decide how they are going to act, and, having acted, how they are going to cope with the results. Perhaps the worst aspect is that even if they maintain the status quo, they get no satisfaction from having done their best, because the patient is manifestly and chronically distressed.

The question of intractable mental pain has to be addressed. We have in health care gone some considerable way with physical illness towards a consensus position about when to allow a person to die; it might be the time to ask whether there is a parallel in mental illness. Given the nature of mental illness it is all the more imperative that we stress at the outset that it is voluntary euthanasia that is the issue here.

This brings us to the wider issue of planned rational euthanasia as propounded by the Voluntary Euthanasia Society. Where do nurses stand in this debate?

In Holland the scene is changing, and we have no reason not to suppose that the moral position on euthanasia in this country may one day shift. Ethical stances do not change overnight, but everyday experiences which cause individuals to question the rights and wrongs of what they are doing or being asked to do, feed into the broader decisions.

AREAS FOR DISCUSSION

- Can individual conscience inform professional decision-making?
- How do nurses cope when patients do not want the care we feel duty bound to give?
- Should nurses be involved in the euthanasia debate?

NOTES AND REFERENCES

1. A. V. Campbell, *Moral Dilemmas in Medicine*, 3rd edn (Edinburgh: Churchill Livingstone, 1984).
2. J. Butler, *Fifteen Sermons*, ed. T. A. Roberts (First published 1726) (London: SPCK, 1970).
3. Thomas Aquinas, *Summa Theologica*.
4. A. Kenny, *Aquinas* (Oxford University Press, 1980).
5. R. Scruton, *A Short History of Modern Philosophy: from Descartes to Wittgenstein* (London: ARK Paperbacks, 1984).
6. A. T. Altschul, 'There won't be a next time', in V. Rippere, R. Williams, (eds.) *Wounded Healers* (Chichester: John Wiley & Son, 1985).

9

AN
EASY DEATH?

Euthanasia is a vast topic – so vast that it is difficult to grasp its full implications. Yet, at the same time it has become a familiar subject, often treated in a matter of fact sort of way.

Euthanasia literally means 'good' or 'easy' death. It has, though, taken on a more sinister tone and conjures up notions of putting to death. Even if we are unhappy at the thought of someone having to lead an impossibly miserable life – be it through pain or disability – to push the sentiment to the point of action is too much for many people to contemplate.

We could mount an argument which says that health care professionals need to have nothing to do with euthanasia in any guise. Thus, while it may be in the interests of the patient to end his life it could be argued that there is no reason why medicine and nursing should become involved. However, this argument is unlikely to stand up to much scrutiny.

It is interesting to compare euthanasia in this context with abortion. There, the medical profession became involved at least in part, because the alternative back-street practice did more harm than a properly run abortion service. One could foresee a similar situation in the field of euthanasia. Like it or not, health professionals are obliged at least to consider their position on euthanasia.

One common response is to reject the notion outright, particularly when it comes with a bald 'euthanasia' tag. There are good reasons for this. Patients could become very nervous if they felt doctors or nurses had become licensed merchants of death, and it is this kind of public reaction which has helped to defeat attempts at legalising voluntary euthanasia.

We have to be very clear about what we mean by euthanasia, and in particular to distinguish between voluntary and imposed euthanasia. A further distinction can be made in imposed euthanasia between involuntary, where the patient could be consulted but is not, and non-voluntary, where the patient cannot be consulted, for instance, in the case of a very young child (Figure 1).

It is worth noting that the British Medical Association *Handbook of Medical Ethics*[1] does not make this distinction. Rather, it talks of 'compulsory euthanasia' – which it defines as 'a decision by society that an individual, either against his will, or without being able to consent, should have his life terminated'. The handbook says that the literal meaning of euthanasia 'carries no ethical difficulties for a doctor, indeed the doctor has a responsibility to ensure that his patient dies with dignity and as little suffering as possible'.

However, the handbook notes that the word euthanasia has been complicated by its interpretation as 'mercy killing' and concludes that 'doctors vary in their approach to passive euthanasia but the profession condemns legalised active euthanasia'. Once again society has to choose between having a legal position on such a complex and emotionally charged matter or leaving itself in the hands of the medical profession which exercises benevolent paternalism. A difficult choice.

Another distinction then is between 'passive' and 'active' euthanasia (Figure 2).

Passive euthanasia is the term used when someone is deliberately allowed to die whereas active euthanasia, as the term suggests, involves an action taken in order to bring about someone's death. Much of the debate on this issue centres on whether or not there is a moral distinction between the two.

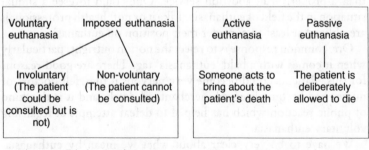

Figure 1. Distinction between different types of euthanasia

Figure 2. Distinction between means of achieving euthanasia

Let us first consider what possible situations would fall into which category. Campbell[2] discusses three types of circumstance in which passive euthanasia, or letting die, is most likely to occur. These are during emergency resuscitation after cardiac arrest; in the case of untreated pneumonia in the severely brain damaged or the terminally ill; and when there is a question over continuation of life support for the severely brain damaged.

In the first two examples we might argue that clinical judgement following the rules of beneficence and non-maleficence should suffice. In the third category where switching off machines or discontinuing feeding is the issue we are perhaps more properly on the ground of euthanasia. Indeed, unless there are sound clinical reasons for such action and the decision is taken within the dictates of the principles of beneficence we are moving towards active non-voluntary euthanasia.

It is perhaps unhelpful to consider cases of passive euthanasia, where the patient is 'allowed to die' without undue medical intervention, under the euthanasia banner, albeit qualified by the label 'passive', for it raises more concerns than are perhaps necessary. Such treatment comes within the principles of beneficence and non-maleficence, and to introduce the notion of euthanasia and its 'putting to death' connotations complicates the business in an unhelpful way.

Active euthanasia is more of a problem for health professionals. A request for voluntary active euthanasia puts a strain on doctors and nurses and goes beyond what they would regard as their job. However, when we are dealing with the terminally ill in considerable pain, or the severely disabled who ask for a way out, drawing the boundaries is less easy. If you hasten death by administering opiates you move from the realms of 'letting die' to active euthanasia – the problem really lies in the grey area in between.

Roman Catholic theologians and philosophers have a doctrine which attempts to deal with this – it is called the doctrine of double effect. This distinguishes between what we do and what we intend the outcome to be. In the case of severe pain in the terminally ill then, if the intention is first to relieve pain and not to kill the patient, we would not be responsible in the same way for the second effect (killing the patient) even if it was foreseen. Our responsibility would then be different from say a deliberate act of murder. The double effect argument does not solve the dilemma but it may help us to cope with it[3].

Yet there are other difficulties. Consider the patient who claims his right to be put to death because his disabilities make his life unbearable. If we accept that as a right, could we also make a case for taking a similar decision for a handicapped neonate, or a severely brain damaged adult? If it was right to kill with permission would it also be right to impose the same 'treatment' where the patient is unable to give consent? If society's answer to this question is yes, then *de facto* it has taken on board non-voluntary euthanasia.

Lorber[4], in a paper on the ethical problems in the management of myelomeningocele and hydrocephalus, argues strongly against such non-voluntary active euthanasia for babies and children who cannot give their considered consent. 'It would be impossible to formulate legislation for it, however humane are the intentions, that could not be abused by the unscrupulous.'

This is a classic statement of the slippery slope argument, the most common and compelling argument against euthanasia, aside from a generalised appeal to the natural law. In its simplest form, the slippery slope argument says that once we embark upon a particular course of action it will possibly lead to an unintended and undesirable state of affairs. In the case of euthanasia, if we accept that there are occasions where killing is the right thing to do, this will somehow, so the argument goes, undermine the moral principles which protect the right to life.

Beauchamp and Childress[5] say that we have to be clear what is encompassed by slippery slope or wedge (as in 'thin end of') arguments. One form of the wedge argument focuses on moral reasoning and the logic of distinctions between different acts. So that if we argue that one course of action is right it will have logical implications for another sort of act that we would generally consider to be wrong. The example that Beauchamp and Childress cite is an abortion which if it is deemed to be right in one set of circumstances may logically imply justification of infanticide in another. This argument rests on Kantian ideas of universalisability, which demands that relevantly similar cases be treated in a similar way. If a severely damaged foetus should be aborted, then a severely damaged baby should be killed.

Beauchamp and Childress draw on Ramsey's[6] work. He argues that ethical and legal mistakes repeat themselves because of this universalisability argument. Ramsay says, 'it is quite clear that at the point of medical, legal and ethical intersections at the edges of life . . . the so-called wedge argument is an excellent one. This is true because legal principles and precedents are systematically designed to apply to other cases as well. This is the way the law "works" and . . . also the way moral reasoning "works" from case to similar case'. Beauchamp and Childress say that 'if we justify the killing of innocent people in medical settings, there is no logical way, according to some arguments, to limit the killing to legitimate cases, for the principle of non-maleficence and the rule against directly killing innocent life have been eroded'. They point out that this version of the wedge argument is not perhaps so compelling as those who use it to uphold distinctions between killing and letting die would like to believe. It can, say Beauchamp and Childress, be used the other way around, that is to argue that there is little moral difference between deliberately killing someone and allowing them to die. They say 'if it is defensible, rationally and morally to allow patients to die under certain conditions, it is rational and morally defensible to kill them under the same conditions'. In other words, if death is in the best interests of the person it is of no relevance how the death comes about.

Harris[7] argues that non-voluntary euthanasia should be legalised. He says that whereas involuntary euthanasia will always be wrong, non-voluntary euthanasia (where the individual's consent cannot be obtained) 'will not be wrong if we are certain that the individual concerned would prefer to die rather than go on living'.

The move from considering passive to active euthanasia tends to begin around the issue of pain relief but this is not where it ends. If nurses and doctors acquired a mandate to kill their patients under certain circumstances, how far would it extend? What about mental pain? What about those patients with restricted physical ability? AIDS patients? What about the socially deprived, those living in intolerable conditions, those who have failed in life? What do we do if these people claim a right to have their lives ended.

We started out by asking whether nurses should have anything to do with euthanasia. In this book we have made a case for the existence of nursing ethics as distinct from medical ethics. This case rests in part on the fact that the same ethical issues will present in different ways for nursing and medicine. Euthanasia is a case in point. Aside from the relatively rare instances of nurses being asked directly if they will assist a patient in taking his life, the main issues in euthanasia confront medicine. This is in large part owing to the fact that any moves towards legalised active euthanasia will involve medicine.

However, nurses are already involved in a day-to-day fashion insofar as they care for the patients who are being 'allowed to die'. Perhaps the most dramatic example of this is the so-called Johns Hopkins[8] case of an infant with Down's syndrome and a digestive tract blockage. The parents refused surgery and the baby was left without treatment. No attempt was made to feed the baby nor was there any attempt to challenge in court the decision to let him die.

It took 15 days for the baby to die. One of the questions the case raises is – should that baby have been killed or left to die? Fifteen days is a long time for nurses to be around an unfed dying infant. The handling of the feelings and emotions involved is no easy matter.

Involuntary active euthanasia is on the face of it unthinkable. But what of the severely brain damaged on life support machines? Kuhse and Singer[8] have a pertinent comment here: 'it is one thing to say, before a life has properly begun, that such a life should not be lived; it is quite different to say that, once a life is being lived, we need not do our best to improve it. We are sometimes prepared to say the former: we are never prepared to say the latter'.

It is in this area that the concept of a living will[9] comes into its own. There has been an increasing tendency in the USA to turn to the legal profession and the most publicised examples of legal involvement in medical treatment to emerge have to do with discontinuation of life support machines, for instance the now famous case of the late Karen Quinlan, and the heroic treatment of handicapped neonates.

A living will is a written statement which people can make before they are ill stating that they do not want life-prolonging treatment should they develop a condition which will result in a poor quality of life. Living wills are clearly intended to serve the interests of the patient, but their operation is not without problems. Alongside the living will there are 'natural death acts' in operation in many States in America. These provide doctors with a constitutional right to refuse life sustaining treatment. The critics of living wills say that there are problems of interpretation as there is a tendency towards vagueness and patients may not have anticipated actual circumstances that occur.

If active euthanasia were ever legalised (a remote possibility as things stand), nurses would be involved. We have been provided with a sample of what that might be like through the work of Dr Peiter Admiraal in Holland – he works with a team of doctors, nurses and a priest. In a report in the *Sunday Times*[10], he gave the impression of being a member of a sensitive team providing good care, reminiscent of the hospice environment. The detailed discussion of the pharmacology involved was rather chilling, yet in all, Admiraal sounds like a caring and moral doctor.

I would, however, sound a note of caution. Although his practice sounds fine (rather as Michel Odent's obstetric practices have their appeal), he is probably the exception. In Admiraal's hands it works, but to transfer his ideas to other practitioners through legislation could well be the start of a slippery slope, and for a nurse working on that slope it could be very difficult indeed.

AREAS FOR DISCUSSION

- Do you think there is a difference between letting die and killing?
- Do you think there is a role for nurses in euthanasia?
- Is the term passive euthanasia a useful one or does it, by introducing the notion of euthanasia into beneficent care, raise more concerns than are necessary?
- Do discussions of euthanasia lead to more harm than good?

NOTES AND REFERENCES

1. British Medical Association. *The Handbook of Medical Ethics* (London: BMA, 1984).
2. A. V. Campbell, *Moral Dilemmas in Medicine*, 3rd edn (Edinburgh: Churchill Livingstone, 1984).
3. I. E. Thompson, K. M. Melia, K. M. Boyd, *Nursing Ethics* (Edinburgh: Churchill Livingstone, 1983).
4. J. Lorber, 'Ethical problems in the management of myelomeningocele and hydrocephalus', *Journal of the Royal College of Physicians*, 10 (1975) 53–8, also cited in ref. 8.
5. T. L. Beauchamp, J. F. Childress, *Principles of Biomedical Ethics*, 2nd edn (Oxford University Press, 1983).
6. P. Ramsey, *Ethics at the edges of life* (New Haven: Yale University Press, 1978).
7. J. Harris, *The Value of Life: an introduction to medical ethics* (London: Routledge and Kegan Paul, 1985).

8. H. Kuhse, P. Singer, *Should the Baby Live? The problem of handicapped infants* (Oxford University Press, 1985).
9. Institute of Medical Ethics, 'Living Wills and the right to refuse treatment', *IME Bulletin*, Supplement no. 5 (1987) pp. 1–6.
10. *Sunday Times Magazine*, June 7, 1987.

10

ACTS OF FAITH

Freedom of information is important in any walk of life, and health care is no exception. We all debate how much patients should be told about their condition. Health professionals have to consider where to draw the line between full disclosure, which is the patient's right, and withholding certain information on the assumption that to disclose would not be in the patient's interests.

These dilemmas address issues of beneficence, non-maleficence, respect for persons and the duty of care. However, there is one other consideration which may not be too comfortable to confront, namely paternalism. That is where health care professionals make choices about the treatment of patients or clients which they deem to be in those clients' best interests.

As we have already seen we have to accept uncertainty as a part of our professional lives. We do not always know until after the event, or sometimes not at all, whether patients would have opted for the same course of action, had they been able to make the choice for themselves.

We often have to act on others' behalf because they are unable to have charge of their own lives. Nurses may take on this responsibility, known as fiduciary responsibility[1], when nursing children, those with a mental illness, unconscious patients or when a patient himself decides to put himself into the hands of his carers.

It is important here to realise that the relationship between nurse (or doctor) and patient is largely based on trust rather than law. Mason and McCall Smith[2] argue that 'what the law expects of the doctor may mirror closely what codes of medical ethics expect, but the basis of compliance in each case is essentially different. Trust and respect are more likely to flourish in a relationship which is governed by morality than by legal rules. The injection of formality with excessive caution into the relationship between doctor and patient is ultimately not in the patient's interests if it means that each sees the other as a potential adversary.' This applies equally to nursing.

Children provide an interesting example of this fiduciary care, and one that is complicated by parents who raise fundamental questions such as who should have the ultimate say in what happens to children. Should parents be deferred to or should children be treated as individuals whose rights must be protected, irrespective of their parents' views? Of course, parents routinely give proxy consent for the treatment of their children, but proxy consents are of real value only if the patient has given authority to the person who consents. If the proxy is thought to be acting unreasonably, then health care staff may override the decision; although, as Mason and McCall Smith point out, this 'would be a hazardous course to adopt'.

Children may be viewed as the property of their parents, or they may be seen as the future workforce and, in some sense, the property of the state. A liberal society tends to give parents more rights in the upbringing of their children although, paradoxically, this limits the children's rights. A more interventionist state approach liberates children and restricts parents[3].

If they are able, patients should give 'informed consent' to treatment. Superficially, informed consent is straightforward enough. Tell the patient what is proposed and, if he agrees, proceed. The principles of informed consent require us to instruct the patient about the ratio of risks and benefits involved in the treatment when compared with alternative treatments or no treatment at all[4,5]. All this does not, of course, cover situations in which he is not able to give consent.

Hence the main principle underlying informed consent is autonomy. Patients must be able to determine what happens to them and make decisions about their treatment. For this to work, patients have to be 'competent' to make judgements and must be given the information required to make them.

The idea of patient competence is difficult and controversial, but it is the question of how much information to disclose that is probably the most vexed. English law allows doctors to determine how much to tell patients when they are attempting to gain their informed consent. This was reaffirmed recently by the Law Lords in the case of Mrs Sidaway[6], who went to court after she had

CASE STUDIES

1 Mrs Johnson gave birth to a boy with considerable spinal deformity. There was some uncertainty about the extent of neurological damage. Mr and Mrs Johnson were asked for their consent to surgical treatment, which would involve a series of operations. One of the surgeons was working on a particular technique with such babies and was having some success, but he also had had some failures. Mrs Johnson decided to ask the nurses what she and her husband should do. The nurses felt torn because they could see the long term gains for future cases and possibly even for the little boy in question, yet they also knew that the treatment was experimental and that the parents were not being told about this aspect.

2 There is major interest in diet and behaviour in a paediatric unit where many hyperactive children are admitted and take part in various randomised trials. The nurses in the unit become concerned as to whether the parents understand when they consent that there may be no direct benefit to their child. Parents are looking for a cure and may not realise that they are allowing their children to be research subjects.

3 Alan Jones was admitted for routine minor surgery. He met the criteria for a randomised control trial which was being carried out at the hospital. The trial had nothing to do with Alan's condition, but researchers simply required a control group. The trial was coming to an end and only a few more cases were required. Although Alan's involvement would have entailed no more than measuring his skull and weighing him, his parents refused to allow him to be used in the research. The staff felt that 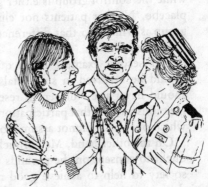 they were being unnecessarily difficult and found it hard to restrain themselves from being over-persuasive.

suffered nerve damage following surgery which, she claimed, she would not have consented to, had she been aware of the risks involved. The Law Lords concluded that 'at the end of the day the doctor, bearing in mind the best interests of the patient, and bearing in mind the patient's right to information which will enable the patient to give a balanced judgement, must decide what information should be given to the patient and in what terms that information should be couched.'

Where does the nurse stand in all this? Mrs Johnson's case raises the question of what counts as research. How do we (or should we) distinguish between experimentation, in the sense of official research, and the development of new treatments, like a new surgical procedure. The Declaration of Helsinki[7], which provides ethical guidelines for involving human beings in research, states that 'in the treatment of a sick person the doctor must be free to use a new diagnostic and therapeutic measure if in his or her judgement it offers hope of saving life, re-establishing health or alleviating suffering'.

Clinical research usually conjures up images of randomised control trials, often, but not invariably, involving drugs. Clinical trials are designed to find out whether a new treatment is better than existing treatments, or no treatment. In blind trials this is achieved by dividing patients into two groups, which, as far as possible, are identical. The experimental group is given the treatment while the control group is either given the standard treatment or a placebo. Neither patients nor clinical staff involved know which group is which, so that differences in outcomes can be attributed to the treatment.

Our second example raises questions about whether children should be involved in such trials at all. Ramsey[8] argues that we should never use children in research because they are unable to give consent, and that participation in research is a matter of altruism which one party cannot assume for another.

On the other hand, McCormick[9] argues that adults and children ought to consent on the grounds that it is to the common good of society to help to achieve good medical care. McCormick argues that parents can consent where the child ought to consent if he or she could.

For adults, at least, the argument is clearer cut. It is obvious that, in order to achieve effective and safe treatment, it is necessary to subject a proportion of the population to some risk. The justification for this is that we have some responsibility towards our fellow men. If we demand safe and beneficial treatment for ourselves we must expect to be at least candidates for clinical research.

The Helsinki Declaration recognises two forms of medical research which involve human subjects: therapeutic research, which will or may benefit the patient directly, and non-therapeutic research which does not. It includes the statement: 'Every biomedical research project involving human subjects should be preceded by careful assessment of predictable risks in comparison with foreseeable benefits to the subject or to others. Concern for the interests of the subject must always prevail over the interests of science and society.'

Mason and McCall Smith[2] describe four types of experimental subjects – individual patients, a group of patients who are suffering from one particular condition, patients who have no association with the disease or process under review but who are readily available, and healthy volunteers.

The hyperactive children in our second example fall into the second group and their position is rather better safeguarded than the handicapped neonate's in the first case. 'Real' research comes under scrutiny, whereas the development of treatments is left more in the hands of the medical profession.

Our third example shows how important it is to be clear about care roles and research roles. In this instance, the patient (or his parents by proxy) has to be sure that his or her interests will come first in any decisions that are made about care.

Nicholson and his colleagues[10] recommend 'that research requiring children as subjects should not be undertaken unless there is a specific and demonstrable need to perform the research on children, and no other route to the relevant knowledge is available'. They suggest that there should be a limit on the number of times that an innovative therapy can be used without submitting it as a formal research project to an ethics committee. And they propose that 'parents and guardians should be considered as trustees of a child's interests, rather than as having rights over the child'. They say that the prime consideration in any research involving children should be that it is not against the interests of any individual child.

Informed consent strikes at the centre of both the art and science of nursing practice. It is required if nursing knowledge is to be advanced, yet its very requirement threatens to jeopardise the trust on which patient–professional relationships are based.

AREAS FOR DISCUSSION

- Children cannot claim their autonomy. Who might serve the best interests of the child: professionals or parents?
- How much information should nurses give to patients about the status of their treatment?
- Is there any social obligation to be involved in research?
- Do you think that children should become involved in research projects?

NOTES AND REFERENCES

1. I. E. Thompson, K. M. Melia, K. M. Boyd, *Nursing Ethics* (Edinburgh: Churchill Livingstone, 1983).
2. J. K. Mason, R. A. McCall Smith, *Law and Medical Ethics* (London: Butterworths, 1987).
3. R. Dingwall, J. Eekelar, T. Murray, *The Protection of Children* (London: Blackwell, 1983).
4. M. D. Kirby, 'Informed consent: what does it mean?' *Journal of Medical Ethics*, 9 (1983) 69–75.
5. V. Herbert, 'Informed consent – a legal evaluation': *Cancer* 46: 4 (1980) 1042–3.
6. Sidaway vs. Board of Governors, Bethlem Royal Hospital (1984)
7. Declaration of Helsinki 1964, revised 1975, in T. L. Beauchamp, J. F. Childress, *Principles of Biomedical Ethics*, 2nd edn (Oxford University Press, 1983).
8. P. Ramsey, *The Patient as Person* (Newhaven: Yale University Press, 1970).
9. R. McCormick, *Experimentation in children: sharing in sociality* (New York: Hastings Centre, 1976).
10. R. H. Nicholson, (ed), *Medical Research with Children: ethics, law and practice*, Institute of Medical Ethics Research Report (Oxford University Press, 1986).

11

TO TELL OR
NOT TO TELL

Confidentiality is very much a topic of the 1980s. We have already examined patients' rights and the rights of health care staff. Rapid developments in information technology have made the public aware that detailed information may be held about them. The Data Protection Act has seen to that, although in fact that act only gives us some safeguards when data are held in computerised form. It is hoped that the spirit of the act will spill over into other kinds of record keeping, but clearly alternative kinds of records will be potentially the most interesting if they are the ones to which the individual has no right of access.

Alongside information technology developments, health care has moved towards a team approach to care and recognition of the social and environmental aspects of health. This means that several professionals or agencies may be involved in the care of an individual patient and that there will be a great amount of information stored about each person. Computerised records are often stored in database form which makes it at least technically possible to link them with other databases such as credit ratings, Inland Revenue and insurance data.

So where do nurses come into the picture? If we consider the notion of privacy and the nature of hospital life, the answer to that question becomes evident. Consider, for example, the matter of history taking. The patient provides a great deal of information about himself, which, if it were not for being in hospital, he would doubtless keep to himself. This could be said to be particularly true in the case of a psychiatric history. The United Kingdom Central Council for Nursing, Midwifery and Health Visiting's code of professional conduct[1] states that the registered nurse shall 'respect confidential information obtained in the course of professional practice and refrain from disclosing such information without the consent of the patient/client or a person entitled to act upon his/her behalf, except where disclosure is required by law or by the order of a court or is necessary in the public interest'.

The UKCC advisory document[2] which elaborates on clause 9 of the code of professional conduct makes it plain that breaches of confidence should be regarded as exceptional. It is worth noting too that despite all the guidelines that are available to nurses the responsibility for breaking a confidence or refusing to disclose confidential information rests with the individual nurse.

Some indication of the legal position is contained in *Guidelines on Confidentiality in Nursing*[3] which states that nurses must not disclose patients' confidences unless there is a lawful excuse which would allow such a breach.

A lawful excuse would be either legal compulsion or patient consent. The guidelines go on to say that patient's rights to confidentiality may be overridden in certain circumstances, namely, 'where the client's own life may be in danger, where there is serious danger to other people, where there is serious threat to the nurse, where there is serious threat to the community, in other circumstances, judged to be exceptional, on the basis of professional consideration and consultation'.

This last condition is clearly open to wide interpretation. However, it is generally true to say that patients expect that their privacy will be respected and so an explicit request for secrecy on the part of the patient might not be held to be necessary.

All this might lead us to ask why it is considered to be a moral thing to do, to keep other people's secrets. At a very general level we would probably all agree that society must operate on the expectation of some trust and honesty. This is especially true in the case of professionals. Society puts its trust in professionals in the expectation that they will respond by acting in an honest and efficient manner. Professionals are by and large, left to regulate their own practice and draw up their own codes of conduct precisely because society feels that it can trust the professions to do this.

However, the basic philosophical question remains – why is it a good thing to keep secrets? Is it that patients will be cared for more effectively if secrets are kept?

The idea of confidentiality is embodied in the Hippocratic Oath: 'Whatever in connection with my professional practice, or not in connection with it, I see or hear in the life of men; which ought

CASE STUDIES

1 A young man is in hospital for investigations of a neurological condition and multiple sclerosis is diagnosed. At visiting time the staff nurse makes some remark to the man's fiancée about his mood and says that it is not surprising in the light of the diagnosis. The man had not told his fiancée because he was not sure how she would react, he had decided to wait a while. After visiting time the patient was extremely angry with the staff nurse and accused her of being unprofessional. The staff nurse had assumed that the fiancée knew the situation and did not think that she had broken any rules of confidentiality.

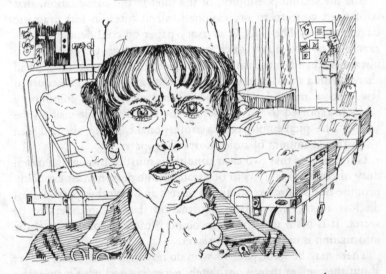

2 A young man is admitted to an accident and emergency department after a road accident. He is not seriously injured and is discharged home a few days later. However, during the admission procedures the staff nurse discovers that he has hard drugs in his possession. She decides not to say anything about it, but subsequently is worried about her decision. The staff nurse made the decision not to say anything on the basis that had the man not been involved in an accident she would not have known about the drugs and so felt that it was somehow unfair to inform the police. On the other hand, she knew the health and social consequences of drug abuse and felt that she had not done her duty to society.

not to be spoken of abroad, I will not divulge, as reckoning that all should be kept secret'.

Gillon[4] puts this question rather neatly when he says: 'essentially medical confidentiality is the respecting of other people's secrets (in the sense of information they do not wish to have further disclosed without their permission). There is obviously no general moral duty to respect other people's secrets (imagine a thief whom one had surprised saying, "shh, don't tell the police, it's a secret"), yet equally obviously doctors, (and, of course other groups) voluntarily undertake some general commitment to keep their patients' or clients' secrets (imagine the same thief talking about his activities in the course of a medical consultation)'.

It is the second possibility, of the thief in the consultation, that is of most concern to professionals, albeit often in less dramatic circumstances. The UKCC advisory paper on confidentiality cites examples of occasions which have caused nurses to worry. Two instances are: a health visitor who realised that information she had shared with a social worker had been used as evidence in a court of law, and a medical practitioner, concerned that a community midwife reported to her employers the fact that while visiting the wife of a hospital employee in a professional capacity, she had seen a substantial amount of stolen hospital property.

Gillon argues that two clear conditions must be present if a moral duty of confidentiality is to be created. One person must explicitly promise not to disclose another's secrets and the other person must disclose to the first person information that he considers to be secret. It is plain that there can be no breach of confidence if the information is not regarded as secret.

There may be some patients who do not wish to reveal any more about themselves than is absolutely necessary and who may prefer that information is handled on a need-to-know basis rather than having a situation where all those who come into contact with the patient are privy to all the available information. There is something of an inverse relationship between the individualisation of care and the assurance of privacy. The problem lies in tailoring care to suit the individual patient's needs, when we have to know quite a bit about the patient. This, with the number of professionals involved, means that the possibility of a breach of confidence is greater.

Bok[5] says that confidentiality refers to the boundaries surrounding shared secrets and to the process of guarding these boundaries. She goes on to say that 'while confidentiality protects much that is not in fact secret, personal secrets lie at its core'.

The UKCC document couches this difficult matter in these terms: 'confidentiality is a rule with certain exceptions. . . . It is essential that before determining that a particular set of circumstances constitute such an exception, the practitioner must be satisfied that the best interests of the patient/client are served thereby or the wider public interest necessitates disclosure'.

UKCC guidelines on confidentiality and the British Medical Association's *Handbook of Medical Ethics*[6] both state that confidentiality is not an absolute principle and say that in exceptional circumstances nurses and doctors might break the rules of confidentiality. The justifications given relate to the patient's best interests, legal requirement and, on occasion, when the public interest overrides the duty of confidentiality.

Guidelines are of necessity rather general in their tone, so professional judgement is very much a matter of each professional deciding whether to tell or not to tell.

Keeping people's secrets can be justified on at least two general philosophical grounds: utilitarian principles and respect for people's autonomy. It is worth taking time to consider these grounds for keeping secrets. The utilitarian argument is clear. In general it states that if patients know that a health care professional will not divulge personal information, then they are more likely to give medical and nursing staff a full account of their condition and circumstances. It is generally presumed that the best possible care will be the result of this medical *glasnost*.

The consequence for society is that patients are not afraid to approach professionals and so the general health of the nation is maintained (and, as Harris[7] wryly points out, professionals remain in work). Harris says that it is often argued that a contract is almost universally assumed by patients. That is to say, patients believe that health care professionals have an obligation to keep their secrets and so have little worry about confiding in staff. In fact medical and nursing confidences do not enjoy legal privilege.

If asked in a court of law, professionals have to 'tell'. It is worth noting, however, as the Royal College of Nursing guidelines make clear, that there is no obligation to disclose information to police officers in many cases in the early stages of an inquiry. The RCN document cites cases of nurses being asked by police for information about patients in accident and emergency departments, or about psychiatric patients. There is clearly a fine distinction to be drawn between protecting a patient's privacy and impeding the course of justice.

With these justifications in mind, it is easy to see where individual situations give rise for concern. General principles are fine until we are confronted with a real life situation which, as ever, is far messier than ethical theories prepare us for. The staff in heart transplantation units are exercised over the issue of confidentiality in domino heart lung transplants where there is a live donor being nursed in the same unit as the recipient. (The recipient of the heart and lungs is the donor for the heart transplant.) The staff work on the premise that the relationship between the patients is best left undisclosed because of the possible detrimental effects upon one or other patient if either of them deteriorates or dies. On the other hand, patients are curious and on occasion have realised whose heart they have. This opens up a whole new debate about the extent to which health care professionals can or indeed should protect their patients from the far-reaching consequences of medical technology.

Sometimes health care workers will want to disclose information which in general would be considered confidential. Again, this has to be a matter of professional judgement which will be as much moral as clinical. The ruling of the BMA about disclosing the results of HIV testing is a case in point. The BMA concluded that doctors should inform the patient's partner when the HIV test result is positive. Doctors are advised to inform the patient and to seek consent to disclosure, but if this is not forthcoming the doctor is obliged to tell the partner in the best interests of that person and the community as a whole.

As society becomes more complex and medical technology advances, the need for privacy and the opportunities for its invasion will grow apace. Nurses, by virtue of their role in society and the trust that is placed in them, will have to maintain an active interest in the business of confidentiality. For it is not something that will be resolved by some rule or law. And it will not go away.

AREAS FOR DISCUSSION

- Is there any obligation to keep a secret even though a patient has not specifically requested secrecy?

- Does a nurse's duty as a responsible citizen override her duty to her patient?
- To what extent should health care professionals withhold information in the interest of protecting a patient?
- What would you do if a patient: confided to you that he had abused his child; or was wanted by the police; or had just been involved in a hit and run accident?

NOTES AND REFERENCES

1. UKCC, *Code of Professional Conduct for the Nurse, Midwife and Health Visitor* (2nd edn) (London: UKCC, 1984).
2. UKCC, *Confidentiality: An elaboration of Clause 9 of the Second Edition of the UKCC's Code of Professional Conduct for the Nurse Midwife and Health Visitor* (London: UKCC, 1987).
3. RCN, *Guidelines on Confidentiality in Nursing* (London: RCN, 1980).
4. R. Gillon, *Philosophical Medical Ethics* (London: John Wiley, 1986).
5. S. Bok, *Secrets: Concealment and Revelation* (Oxford University Press, 1986).
6. BMA, *The Handbook of Medical Ethics* (London: BMA, 1984).
7. J. Harris, *The Value of Life: an introduction to medical ethics* (London: Routledge and Kegan Paul, 1985).

12

ETHICS IN
CONTEXT

Throughout this book I have tried to present everyday cases and issues which individual nurses may encounter within the context of a wider ethical debate. In clinical practice problems often occur which require action; there is not always time for much deliberation. There is a tendency to look for some kind of guide to reasonable action in these circumstances. On the whole ethical codes are of limited help in this respect. Generalised ethical statements and idealised positions are by their very nature not going to provide a programme for action in all eventualities. All along we have seen that personal and professional morality may be in conflict. Ethical principles often oppose one another. For instance we may wish to uphold the rights of an individual patient only to find that a more generalised notion of justice is being compromised.

On the bottom line we find that ethics is very much bound up with politics. In this last chapter I want to try to pull these ideas together by considering where codes of ethics might play a part, by looking at how the political dimension of health care fits into the debate.

Once we realise that there is a societal aspect to most issues in health care we are some way towards recognising the political dimension. An interesting question to raise, then, is to what extent nurses should be concerned with politics. Some might want to ask the question, can nurses *not* be involved in politics? – depending on its interpretation this can be seen as an ethical question in itself.

The arrival of AIDS presents both a dramatic and an everyday example of how a health issue goes beyond the scope of health care professionals and presents both moral and political problems for society. As the numbers of HIV positive members of the population grow and those who go on to develop the full blown syndrome multiplies, AIDS becomes an everyday fact for increasing numbers of health care workers. Nurses in the community stand an ever growing chance of coming into contact with AIDS patients and their families. Nurses are by and large not prepared for this new and possibly frightening addition to their workload.

It is clear that AIDS presents far more than a health care problem. It challenges society by posing a real threat to health and lifestyle. Perhaps the greatest moral problem for nurses is that they find themselves confronting their own motives, moral perspectives and prejudices. We may blithely say, 'I will care for anyone, whatever their condition, whatever their lifestyle', and then begin to have doubts. The objection to offering unconditional care is expressed in physical terms: Is there a danger? Who comes first – nurses or patients? What about nurses' families? In short, nurses may find themselves asking how far the caring ethic goes. The nursing profession is no more immune from panic, fear and prejudice than any other group in society. Nurses as members of society are part of its response to AIDS, they are neither above it nor apart from it. Nurses are both affected by the societal response and contribute to it.

Medicine too has to face this fact. The General Medical Council saw the need to declare that doctors refusing to treat AIDS patients could face serious misconduct charges. The GMC is reported to have become seriously concerned that some doctors have refused to provide care for sufferers or those who are HIV positive. Uncertainty and ignorance about how the disease spreads has led to much insensitivity towards AIDS patients, and actions have, on occasion, been extreme. The Public Health (Control of Diseases) Act 1984 was amended in 1985 to add AIDS to the list of diseases already covered – typhus, smallpox, cholera and plague. A man was ordered to be compulsorily detained in a Manchester hospital under the provisions of this act[1]. Nursing this patient must have been very difficult. The nurses had to relate to a patient who was being compulsorily detained without any recourse to the usual beneficence arguments that go along with a similar detention order under the Mental Health Act.

The UKCC code of professional conduct[2] states that 'each registered nurse, midwife and health visitor shall act, at all times, in such a manner as to justify public trust and confidence, to uphold and enhance the good standing and reputation of the profession, to serve the interests of society, and above all to safeguard the interests of individual patients and clients'. According to this code it is clear that AIDS patients have as much right to be cared for as any other sick person. Yet the societal response to AIDS has complicated the issue; it has produced categories which come close to Victorian distinctions between the deserving and undeserving poor. In other words the notion of blame has crept in, rendering innocent patients and culpable patients. Nurses have to confront their own personal stance on these issues when they nurse AIDS patients. Among the many viewpoints, the divine vengeance lobby sees an empirical justification for the stance that they take in the demographic fact that the majority of AIDS cases come from sectors of society that are seen by some to be blameworthy.

At the societal level then, we can see how AIDS patients and HIV positive people are in danger of being stigmatised and segregated. Nurses, as individuals, face patients and their symptoms and their feelings, they also face the families and friends of those patients. However, as individuals, nurses also have their own fears and prejudices. A pragmatic approach to accommodating these two factors would place an emphasis on the facts about AIDS rather than the myths, and would allow free discussion among nurses so that they can vent their feelings and somehow sort out their emotive reaction to AIDS and move towards a rational workable approach to patient care. Clearly this is easier to say than to do. This is the essence of the challenge.

A nurse's duty to care is based largely on a contract of trust rather than on a set of legal rules. Perhaps the most pervasive ethical basis for determining the rights and wrongs of nursing actions can be found in the Golden Rule attributed to Moses[3]. This 'do unto others as you would have them do unto you' dictat is a widely held ethical premise. Kantian ethics, with its emphasis on duty and treating others as ends in themselves and not simply as means to ends, stresses the need for respect for persons. AIDS patients require our respect because they form part of what Kant calls the community of moral agents, that is people who behave towards each other according to a basic principle of respect for each other. Respect involves our caring for patients without passing judgement. Whether a patient has AIDS because he shares needles, had casual sex abroad or because he is a haemophiliac receiving transfused blood, should make no difference to the nature of his care.

Yet as we move into the areas of life where morals are closer to the surface, for example sexually transmitted disease, there is more of a tendency to make moral as well as clinical judgements. A moral order is superimposed on the social facts, so that we have 'culpable gays' and 'innocent babies' dying of AIDS.

Codes of ethics can be invoked to protect patients' rights to care. The only area of patient care to date where there is a possibility for staff to opt out of care is abortion. What grounds might health care workers cite to excuse them from caring for AIDS patients? A General Medical Council[4] report on this stated that, 'it is unethical for a doctor to withhold treatment for any patient merely on the grounds that the doctor disapproves of that patient's lifestyle. Also it is inconsistent with the traditions of the medical profession for a doctor to refuse treatment simply because the condition could expose the doctor to personal risk. People have traditionally expected to get help from a doctor even when suffering from the most virulent infection.'

The same argument has been made for nursing. The Royal College of Nursing AIDS guidelines[5] state that it is 'the responsibility of all nurses to offer appropriate and meaningful care to the sick. There is no opt-out clause for caring for patients with AIDS/HIV related diseases, and refusal to care may well result in disciplinary procedures being taken against the nurse for unprofessional conduct'.

The health service has long been a politically important issue, but such is the heat within the debate at the moment it is almost impossible to ignore the political dimension of health care.

As we have seen so far in this book, professional and private morality are issues which have to be addressed in everyday practice. They must also be considered in relation to achieving change. This opens up a much wider debate. What kind of change are we talking about – changing practice, changing policy, changing the government's mind? At different times we could be talking about any or all of these. The question is how legitimate it is for a health care professional group to do this. And what are the moral issues involved in so doing? Clay[6] argues that 'nurses must be able to fight for the changes they want without turning the ward into a battleground'. This is all very well, but whether or not society as a whole wishes to go along with this will surely be contingent upon *what* nurses want to fight for.

Until recently, medical opinion has tended to hold sway, clinical judgement covered a broad area and went largely unquestioned. The government's open quarrel with the BMA in 1988 over National

Health Service funding marks a shift from the long standing acceptance of our paternalistic medical profession. Medicine's right to practise as it sees fit has been called into question. This means that moral positions are being exposed and the problematic and highly political nature of health care decisions becomes evident.

The point I want to address is not whether in the current debates on the NHS the nursing and medical professions or the government was right, but the question of who should say what constitutes health care. In other words, how far does professional judgement go? Where do politics and professional health care work meet?

We are in a sense talking about professional judgement versus budgetary control in the determination of what health care should look like. It is all too easy to allow the politics of health care to drive the clinical perspective. At heart, then, we have a question of power.

When we set some of the everyday ethical issues that nurses face into a wider context, it becomes clear why we have to consider nursing politics as well as nursing ethics. At the same time, it becomes even clearer that we must determine the stance that the profession as a whole wishes to adopt, a stance which will be based on professional judgement and not some kind of position which leaves nurses vulnerable to being used as union fodder in another battle. We have then to tackle the thorny question of the professional and personal values and politics which are involved. To argue that professionals should leave their personal morality outside when they step into health care and adopt instead the professional morality is not only easier said than done, but is a questionable position.

Let us look briefly at the case that might be made for nursing to have a political face. What might constitute a need for nursing politics? What would the mandate look like? Which issues are nurses going to take up – the state of the health service, their own conditions of work, a hearing in the debate? We run immediately into difficulty here as these issues are not altogether separate. It is worth commenting here that the organisation of nursing's professional body is not as helpful as it might be, if only from a public relations viewpoint. Unlike the medical profession, nursing does not have a Royal College which is unconcerned with union activities. This necessarily clutters any professional statement that it might wish to make about patient care needs with self-interested union-style positions. In the case of medicine the Royal Colleges' statements can be made separately from anything that the BMA might wish to propound.

So what of the politics of nursing? A simplistic view on the provision of health care might have it that a health service needs to hire a variety of workers to undertake the various tasks involved and that these workers should perform the work within the overall philosophy and constraints, organisational and budgetary, of the service. Close as this may sound to the position that Roy Griffiths has had us move into, it is too simple a view for several reasons. Professional judgement cannot be invoked as an excuse for extravagance and ill thought out practices which cannot be justified.

The simplistic model will not do. First, it is in the nature of professional work that those undertaking the work have some view on how it should be carried out and indeed what it should comprise. Thus we have professional groups operating according to what Everett Hughes[7] has called licence and mandate. Licence to practice is easily understood. It ensures that there is some sort of control over the kinds of people who are allowed to undertake particular kinds of work. It keeps out the quacks and protects the public, if you will. Mandate is rather more complex. Hughes claims that certain occupations, once they are granted a licence, go on to claim a mandate. Taking medicine as an example, he argues that doctors not only do the work of medicine, but they also determine what shall constitute medical work.

We can see then, that health care amounts to more than a simple matter of having work to do and employing someone to do it, because these doers have claimed a right to determine the nature of the work. Specialised knowledge and skills along with a lengthy training and registration makes it possible for professionals to keep a monopoly on their work. Health care professionals have to be kept in check by society because many of the clinical judgements they make have a moral dimension.

It is perhaps all too easy for professionals to gain a moral as well as a clinical monopoly in health care. It is in large part inevitable and perhaps desirable that nursing and medicine take moral stances in health care, an amoral approach to care of the sick would not be in anyone's interests. It is important, though, that this dimension of health care work is recognised for what it is.

To date it would appear that society has been content to let professionals work out the moral dimension of health care. Medical technological advances have tended to make some ethical issues more public and so we have wide media coverage of *in vitro* fertilisation surrogacy, use of life support systems and transplant surgery. However, even when such major dilemmas are absent there is often some moral question at the heart of a clinical decision. So how do professionals make the distinction, if indeed they do, between their personal moral stance and that of the profession? How they handle this question is crucial. Codes of ethics are of some help, but they are only part of the story. In any case professional codes of ethics do not drop fully formed from the skies; they are written by individuals and based on some collective notion of morality which has drawn upon the individual value systems of the writers of the code.

Professional ethics in nursing, based as it is on principles of beneficence, respect for persons and justice, does not allow us to escape the political aspect of our business. When nurses come to act according to their political convictions they may find that these principles are thrown into confusion. Justice – the demand for universal fairness – may require some limitations on individual patient's rights.

The principle of justice, it could be argued, requires those in the thick of health service work to maintain and if necessary defend standards of care. What if this involves political activity on the part of professional associations? The UKCC code of professional conduct is interesting as it could be said to cut two ways. On the one hand the code can be used as a public sign that nurses can be trusted to behave in a way that will be in the patient's best interests. Patients would not expect to have their care compromised by, say, strike action by the nursing staff. On the other hand, consider Clauses 10 and 11 of the code: 'have regard to the environment of care and its physical, psychological and social effects on patients/clients, and also to the adequacy of resources, and make known to appropriate persons or authorities any circumstances which could place patients/clients in jeopardy or which militate against safe standards of practice' and 'have regard to the workload of and the pressures on professional colleagues and subordinates and take appropriate action if these are seen to be such as to constitute abuse of the individual practitioner and/or to jeopardise safe standards of practice'. These could lead some to the conclusion that some kind of industrial action was appropriate.

Ethics and politics, in the end, come down to individual decisions. Nurses may look to colleagues and codes but ultimately they have to face the uncomfortable fact that their professional judgement has an ethical dimension which may in turn also stir their political considerations. We are often left with the most simple litmus test of all: 'how would I like it if that was me?' Even this 'do as you would be done by' approach is not foolproof. Mackie[8] points this out by referring to Bernard Shaw's comment on the Golden Rule, 'Do not do unto others as you would have that they should do unto you. Their tastes may not be the same'.

Campbell[9] has perhaps the most sanguine yet deeply practical approach to codes of ethics. He says, 'all that a profession can be expected to do is to provide some generalised statements in everyday language and leave it to the good sense and good will of its practitioners to deal with the ambiguous situations. It is the moral philosopher's job to get at the meanings of the seemingly simply terms that we use in ethical debate – "good", "best interests", "respect" etc.'.

Nursing, as we have demonstrated in this book is rife with difficult situations which raise moral issues and call for moral choices to be made. If nurses take the time to look at the choices they make and attempt to justify them, then nursing ethics can develop and establish itself alongside medical ethics. Ethical codes will take us some of the way, but we have to accept that moral uncertainty is part and parcel of nursing practice. It will be the constant awareness of the ethical dimension of nursing along with a serious attempt to keep nursing ethical debate alive that will best lay the foundation of the fast growing entity that is nursing ethics.

NOTES AND REFERENCES

1. General Medical Council statement, *IME Bulletin* No. 26 (London: Institute of Medical Ethics, 1987).
2. UKCC, *Code of Professional Conduct, for the Nurse, Midwife and Health Visitor*, 2nd edn (London: UKCC, 1984).
3. P. Singer, *Practical Ethics* (Cambridge University Press, 1979), p. 9.
4. *IME Bulletin* No. 26 (London: Institute of Medical Ethics, 1987) p. 14.
5. *AIDS Nursing Guidelines* (London: Royal College of Nursing, 1987).
6. T. Clay, *Nurses, Power and Politics* (London: Heinemann, 1987).
7. E. C. Hughes, *Men and their work* (New York: The Free Press of Glencoe, 1957).

8. J. L. Mackie, *Ethics: inventing right and wrong* (Harmondsworth: Penguin Books, 1977).
9. A. V. Campbell, *Moral Dilemmas in Medicine* (Edinburgh: Churchill Livingstone, 1984).

FURTHER READING

1. These books offer a good general introduction to ethics. Mackie's book provides a clear introduction to ethics moving from a discussion of the subjectivity of values to consider the central ideas of moral philosophy. Frankena's work offers a complex yet concise introduction to ethics.

W. K. Frankena, *Ethics* (New Jersey: Prentice Hall, 1973).

R. M. Hare, *The Language of Morals* (Oxford University Press, 1964).

J. L. Mackie (1977) *Ethics: Inventing Right and Wrong* (Harmondsworth: Penguin Books, 1977).

D. D. Raphael, *Moral Philosophy* (Oxford University Press, 1980).

P. Singer, *Practical Ethics* (Cambridge University Press, 1979).

2. These books are essentially concerned with medical ethics. As nursing ethics and medical ethics have much in common, they constitute useful reading for those interested in nursing ethics.

Gillon's book is a good introduction to the area. Veatch's work makes a good reference book. Beauchamp and Childress is rather detailed but has the attraction of an appendix of 35 cases which are constantly drawn upon in the text. It also reproduces a number of the important codes of ethics. Campbell draws quite extensively on cases which involve issues of particular relevance to nursing. Downie and Calman take a useful approach in which they devote the first half of the book to moral philosophy and the second to setting it in a clinical context. This work provides a good basis for ethical debate. Lockwood's work is a collection of papers each devoted to a specific issue or concept.

T. L. Beauchamp, J. L. Childress, *Principles of Biomedical Ethics*, 2nd edn (Oxford University Press, 1983).

A. V. Campbell, *Moral Dilemmas in Medicine*, 3rd edn (Edinburgh: Churchill Livingstone, 1984).

R. S. Downie, K. Calman, *Healthy Respect: ethics in health care* (London: Faber and Faber, 1987).

R. Gillon, *Philosophical Medical Ethics* (London: John Wiley, 1986).

M. Lockwood, ed, *Moral Dilemmas in Modern Medicine* (Oxford University Press, 1985).

R. M. Veatch, *A theory of medical ethics* (New York: Basic Books, 1981).

3. These are specifically nursing ethics books, and while the moral and clinical discussions are often similar to many of those found in the other works, the focus is specifically on nursing ethics.

G. Rumbold, *Ethics in nursing practice* (London: Ballière, 1986).

I. E. Thompson, K. M. Melia, K. M. Boyd, *Nursing ethics*, 2nd edn (Edinburgh: Churchill Livingstone, 1988).

INDEX

AUTHOR INDEX

SUBJECT INDEX